Self-assessm

Derm   ...ology

GM Kavanagh
MB, MRCP
Consultant Dermatologist
Edinburgh Royal Infirmary
Edinburgh
UK

JA Savin
MA, MD, FRCP, DIH
Consultant Dermatologist
Edinburgh Royal Infirmary
Edinburgh
UK

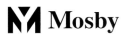 Mosby

London · Philadelphia · St Louis · Sydney · Tokyo

Related titles published in Mosby's Testing series include:

Cardiology
Clinical Dermatology
Clinical Infectious Disease
Clinical Medicine
Clinical Neurology
Clinical Surgery
Ear, Nose and Throat
Embryology, 2nd Edition
Endocrinology, 2nd Edition
Gastroenterology, 2nd Edition
Hematology
Human Histology
Human Anatomy
Hypertension

Infectious Diseases
Injury in Sport
Medicine:
  Vols 1–4
Oral Medicine
Orthopaedics
Otolaryngology
Paediatrics
Pathology
Renal Disease
Rheumatology
Sexually Transmitted Diseases
Urology

Development Editor:	**Gina Almond**
Project Manager:	**Janine Smith**
Production:	**Siobhán Egan**
Index:	**John Gibson**
Design:	**Paul Phillips**
Cover Design:	**Paul Phillips**
Publisher:	**Jane Ryley**

Copyright © 1998 Mosby International Ltd.

Published in 1998 by Mosby, an imprint of Mosby International Ltd.

ISBN 0 7234 2553 1

Printed and bound by Keslan Servicios Gráficos

Contents

1. Weakness and a streaky rash   1

2. Hot legs and a swollen abdomen   7

3. A traveller with diarrhoea   13

4. A man with a grey face   19

5. A rash stroke   24

6. Pain and proteinuria   31

7. Flat and shiny   37

8. Hark the herald!   43

9. Right on target?   49

10. Ulcers and erosions   55

11. A clue from a condom   62

12. Striped nails and a furry tongue   69

13. Persistent skin splinters   75

14. When is a keloid not a keloid?   80

15. Notched nails and a nasty smell   85

16. Rapidly progressive nasal ulceration   91

17. Sunny side up   97

18. A surgical cure of itching   104

19. An ulcer to be kept away from the surgeons   110

20. Pink patches and purple nodules   116

21. Shades of King George   126

22. Psoriasis – or not?   133

23. Feckless and freckled   139

24. Rings and things   144

25. Dangerous swellings   151

Index   156

Preface

We present here the details of a series of patients who have been seen in our clinics recently. The question and answer format is designed to allow readers to test their knowledge first, and then to learn more about each topic.

The conditions described range from the common to the rare, and we hope that this book will be of interest to most doctors and to many senior medical students. Its emphasis on conditions that have internal associations will make it particularly useful to those preparing for a higher qualification in general medicine, and to those, such as general practitioners, who need a good general grasp of dermatology.

GM Kavanagh
JA Savin
May 1998

Acknowledgements

Most of the clinical photographs come from our departmental collections, with the exception of Figs 7.10 and 7.11 which were kindly provided by the Photobiology Unit at St John's Institute of Dermatology, St Thomas' Hospital, Lambeth Palace Road, London. and Figs 1.10 and 1.11 which are reproduced with permission of *Acta-dermatovenerologica*.

We are particularly grateful to Dr K McLaren, University Department of Pathology, Medical School, Edinburgh, for providing many of the hematoxylin and eosin and immunofluorescence pictures.

We are indebted to Dr John W Evans FRACR, Queen Margaret Hospital, Dunfermline, for the provision and expert interpretation of all X-rays and imaging pictures.

Our thanks to Dr George Beveridge, Department of Dermatology, University of Edinburgh, for Figs 3.5 (a and b), Figs 22.9 and 22.10.

Dr D Ho-Yen, Consultant Microbiologist, Raigmore Hospital, Inverness, kindly gave us Figs 24.4 and 24.5.

Thanks to Dr Michael Kramer, Institute of Dermatopathology, Jefferson Medical College, Philadelphia, USA, for Fig. 24.8.

Finally, our thanks also to 'deerest' Alec Keith (Fig. 24.6).

Weakness and a
1 streaky rash

Case History

A 55-year-old man developed a scaly, red rash – mainly on his face, neck, chest and abdomen, and extensor aspects of his limbs (**Figs 1.1–1.3**). It worsened after exposure to the sun, and there was marked periorbital oedema. Over the next 3 weeks he found it increasingly difficult to climb stairs and to lift things above his head.

Examination revealed violaceous streaks on his fingers (**Fig. 1.4**), as well as areas of a similar colour on his elbows, knees, and trunk. Periungal erythema, telangiectasia, and ragged cuticles were also present (**Fig. 1.5**). Initial investigations were carried out and the results are shown in **Fig. 1.6**.

Questions

1. **What is the diagnosis?**
2. **What additional investigations would you perform?**
3. **What complications may arise?**
4. **How should this condition be managed, and what is its prognosis?**

→ Fig. 1.1
Diffuse dusky erythema with swelling of the eyelids. This is typical of this condition.

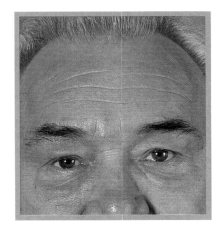

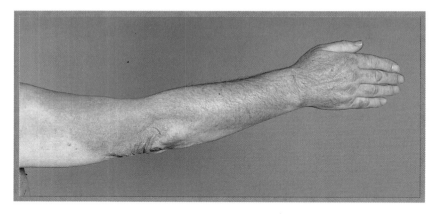

↑ Fig. 1.2
Violaceous erythema in a sun-exposed distribution, with a sharp cut-off.

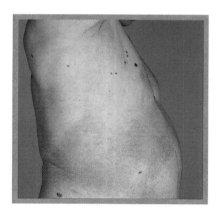

↑ Fig. 1.3
This condition affects not only light-exposed sites but the trunk and buttocks also.

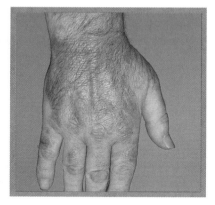

↑ Fig. 1.4
Distinctive streaks of linear dusky erythema running down the backs of the fingers. Gottron's papules are pathognomonic of this condition, lying on the backs of the meta-carpophalangeal joints and finger joints.

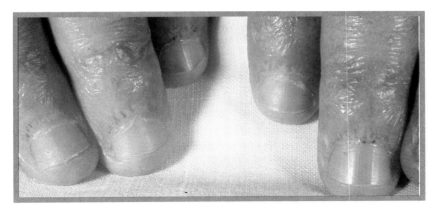

↑ Fig. 1.5
Note the striking telangiectasia of the proximal nail folds and the ragged cuticles.

→Fig. 1.6
Table of initial investigations.

Initial investigations	
FBC, ESR:	Normal
U&E, creatinine, LFTs:	Normal
ANA, immunoglobulins:	Normal

Answers

1. Dermatomyositis (DM). The word 'heliotrope', applied to the changes on the eyelids, refers to the colour of heliotrope plants (**Fig. 1.7**). The facial erythema in DM may be indistinguishable from that of acute cutaneous lupus erythematosus (LE), and DM may form part of an overlap syndrome with other connective diseases such as systemic sclerosis. Periorbital oedema is common in early DM, and has been mistaken for angioedema (see **Fig. 25.5**). The periungal erythema and telangiectasia is typical of, but not specific for, DM (see Case 5), but Gottron's papules on the knuckles are characteristic (see Fig. 1.4).

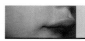

2. Changes in muscle enzyme levels are the most sensitive indicator of disease activity. In particular, creatine phosphokinase (CPK) and aldolase levels are raised in over 95% of patients with DM.

Electromyography is abnormal in about 80% of patients (**Fig. 1.8**). Significant findings include:
• low amplitude, short duration, and polyphasic potentials;
• spontaneous fibrillation;
• increased irritability on the insertion of electrodes;
• positive sharp waves.

Muscle biopsy is abnormal in 90% of patients, but the inflammatory and necrotic changes are focal, and so may be missed. For this reason, magnetic resonance imaging is now the investigation of choice, although is limited by its availability (**Fig. 1.9**).

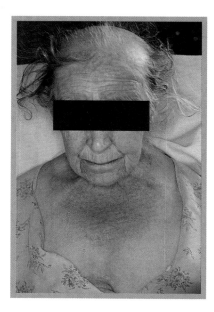

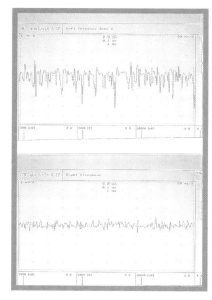

↑ Fig. 1.7
Ironically, this patient with dermatomyositis is wearing a night-dress depicting heliotrope plants, which are typically red–purple in colour and are named for their tendency to turn toward the sun.

↑ Fig. 1.8
The EMG tracing above is normal, while the one below is from a patient with dermatomyositis, and shows low amplitude, polyphasic action potentials.

In this patient, a search for an underlying carcinoma was negative. A 20–50% prevalence of malignancy has been reported in DM. The tumours can appear before, at the same time as, or after the onset of the DM (**Figs 1.10** and **1.11**). There is debate about how hard one should look for an underlying malignancy. However, a careful physical examination, urinalysis, stool sampling for occult blood, a chest X-ray, and ultrasound of the pelvis in females, all seem justifiable in adults.

Several autoantibodies have been described in DM/polymyositis, and are apparently specific for the disease, although they are not detected in most patients. The antibody to histidyl tRNA synthetase (Jo-1) is more common in patients with polymyositis and interstitial lung disease.

A skin biopsy usually shows nonspecific inflammation only. Advanced lesions may be indistinguishable histologically from LE, with epidermal atrophy, liquefaction of the basal layer, and a patchy infiltrate of mononuclear cells.

3. Neck, facial, and pharyngeal muscles may be affected, causing difficulty in swallowing and speaking. Esophageal dysmotility is common – in severe cases, nasogastric feeding is needed to avoid aspiration pneumonia.

Cardiac involvement – with myositis, or a conduction system defect, or both – occurs in most patients with adult DM, and is a relatively common cause of death. Lung disease is also common, and may be due to interstitial fibrosis, aspiration pneumonia, or hypoventilation from weakened respiratory muscles.

Vasculitis is much more common in childhood than in adult DM, and the bowel may be affected, resulting in ulceration, bleeding, and perforation.

Calcinosis of muscles, tendons, or the skin occurs in more than half of childhood cases and in about 15% of affected adults. It is a good prognostic feature. The muscles typically involved are those of the pelvic and shoulder girdles. Calcium may extrude through the skin with ulcers and cellulitis.

→ Fig. 1.9
This fat-suppressed image through the thighs shows an increased signal from the left rectus femoris and quadriceps muscles compared with the adductors. This indicates inflammation in these muscles.

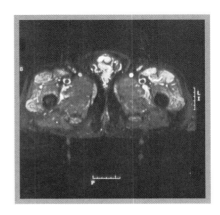

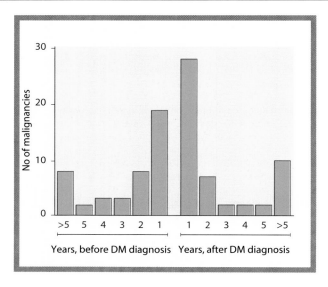

← **Fig. 1.10** Temporal relation of the diagnosis of cancer to that of dermatomyositis.

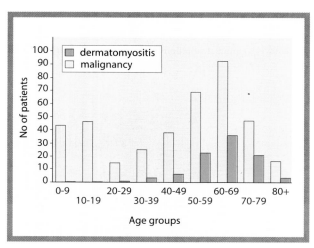

← **Fig. 1.11** This graph shows the increasing association of malignancy with increasing age.

Hot legs and a swollen
2 | abdomen

Case History

A 30-year-old patient known to have been an alcoholic for many years, was admitted with severe upper abdominal pain, fever, and generalised weakness. He had been drinking heavily in binges over the preceding month. On admission he was pale and distressed, with a pyrexia of 39°C and a grossly distended abdomen (**Fig. 2.1**) which showed shifting dullness. A number of investigations, including a CT scan of the abdomen (**Fig. 2.2**), were performed. The results of the other analyses are shown in **Fig. 2.3**.

Within 3 days he developed a blotchy, painful rash on the lower legs, with swelling of the ankles and feet (**Figs 2.4** and **2.5**). A diagnosis was made, and treatment with a specific drug (potassium iodide) was started, but the lesions finally resolved only when his acute abdominal condition settled.

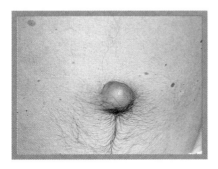

↑Fig. 2.1
Marked abdominal distension, with eversion of the umbilicus.

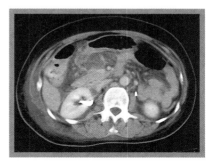

↑Fig. 2.2
This CT scan of the upper abdomen shows a bulky head of pancreas, induration of the adjacent fat planes, and some free fluid around the tip of the liver. These features are typical of pancreatitis, and there is no calcification to indicate chronic pancreatitis.

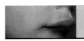

Questions

1. **What diagnosis would explain both the abdominal and skin changes ?**
2. **What changes would you expect to see in a skin biopsy?**
3. **What are the other important causes of this skin condition?**

Investigations	
FBC:	Hb 10.5g/dl, WCC 13.8 × 10⁹/l, platelets normal
Urea:	11.3mmol/l
Sodium:	116mmol/l (normal=132–144mmol/l)
Calcium:	1.7mmol/l (normal=2.1–2.6mmol/l)
LFTs:	γGT 136u/l, alkaline phosphatase 689iu/l, albumin 24g/l
Amylase:	11, 591iu/l (normal=50–300iu/l)

← Fig. 2.3
Table of other investigations.

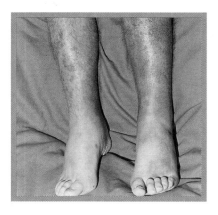 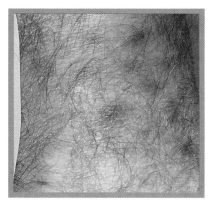

↑Figs 2.4 and 2.5
Distant and close-up views of the blotchy, confluent rash on the lower legs which included scattered smaller purpuric lesions. This rash was hot and painful.

Answers

1. Pancreatic panniculitis (inflammation of the subcutaneous fat), following release of pancreatic enzymes into the peripheral circulation. Neutrophils, attracted to the subcutaneous fat by pancreatic enzymes, cause an extensive necrosis of adipocytes. An association is well recognised between pancreatitis, or pancreatic carcinoma, and erythematous nodules (usually on the lower legs and less commonly on the buttocks and trunk), fever, and also, occasionally, polyserositis. Men are predominantly affected, usually in the fourth to sixth decades.

Subcutaneous fat reacts to a range of insults in a limited number of ways. Panniculitis is the umbrella term for a spectrum of disorders involving adipose tissue. Other than the pancreatic form, they mainly affect women, who are overweight.

Panniculitis is usually classified by its histopathological features, as its pathogenesis is so poorly understood. Traditionally, panniculitides are divided into lobular and septal types, on the basis of the distribution of the inflammatory infiltrate lying either within the lobules of adipocytes or in the surrounding septae (**Fig. 2.6**). These can be further subdivided, according to the presence or absence of vasculitis. In reality, panniculitides seldom fall clearly into either of the two main groups. The exception to this is erythema nodosum, which is classically septal in distribution, if biopsied early. It is difficult, if not impossible, to establish a histological diagnosis without a deep biopsy.

2. The histopathological changes in this form of panniculitis are unique. In the early stages, focal areas of fat necrosis are seen in lobules, especially at their periphery. With time, extensive fat necrosis with a surrounding infiltrate of neutrophils develops, in association with saponification that ranges from slight to severe, with a sparse superficial and deep lymphocytic infiltrate in the dermis. Striking calcification within fat lobules and 'ghost-like' adipocytes may appear in the late stages.

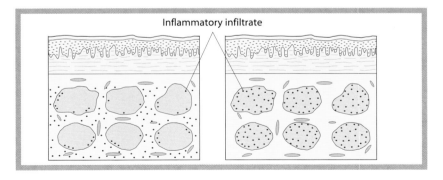

↑ Fig. 2.6
The lobular and septal types of panniculitis: the inflammatory infiltrate on the right lies mainly within the lobules of adipocytes, whereas that on the left is mainly septal.

3. **Erythema nodosum (Fig. 2.7).** This reactive inflammation of the subcutaneous tissue can be associated with a variety of underlying conditions. Ill-defined, tender, erythematous nodules or plaques typically involve the shins, and less frequently the arms. They may be preceded or accompanied by fever, malaise, and arthralgia. Lesions pass through a typical bruise-like phase before resolving without any scarring. Nodules may continue to appear over many weeks, but usually the episode will subside in 3–6 weeks. Many triggering factors exist, including infectious agents (streptococci, yersinia, mycobacteria), drugs (sulfonamides, oestrogen, oral contraceptives), sarcoidosis, and inflammatory bowel disease. However, a definite cause can be found in only about 50% of cases. Treatment is supportive – bed rest and nonsteroidal anti-inflammatory agents. Oral potassium iodide has been used, and systemic steroids – if not contraindicated by an underlying infection – are sometimes necessary .

    Nodular vasculitis (erythema induratum). Tender, erythematous nodules appear on the calves of middle-aged women. The lesions resolve slowly, and have a tendency to recur, and sometimes to ulcerate, if the vasculitis is severe (**Fig. 2.8**). The aetiology is unknown, but the original cases described by Bazin all had tuberculosis. In cases associated with tuberculosis, there may be caseation necrosis and tuberculoid granulomas, but no bacilli can be seen. Histologically, an inflammatory infiltrate is seen throughout the fat lobules, and in septae near involved blood vessels. Deposition of fibrin within large-vessel walls (a hallmark of vasculitis) is typical, and eosinophils are often present.

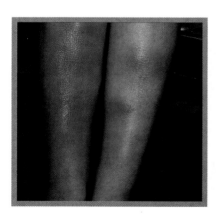

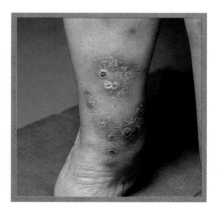

↑ Fig. 2.7
Erythema nodosum: a wide range of drugs, infectious agents, and systemic diseases can cause this reaction pattern.

↑ Fig. 2.8
Erythema induratum: this typically affects middle-aged women, on the back of their calves. Many have a chilblain tendency and puffy ankles.

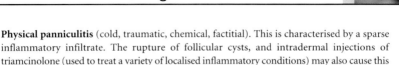
Physical panniculitis (cold, traumatic, chemical, factitial). This is characterised by a sparse inflammatory infiltrate. The rupture of follicular cysts, and intradermal injections of triamcinolone (used to treat a variety of localised inflammatory conditions) may also cause this type of panniculitis. Systemic steroids can also cause panniculitis, but the mechanism is unknown.

Metabolic panniculitis. In α_1-antitrypsin deficiency, an absence of the serum protease inhibitor leads to unopposed tissue breakdown. The most common association is with early, rapidly progressive emphysema, but the condition has also been linked to a variety of systemic diseases. Tender erythematous nodules appear over the trunk and limbs, and, characteristically, ulcerate after minimal trauma. Spontaneous drainage, fever, pleural effusions, and pulmonary emboli are common. Levels of α_1-antitrypsin may be low, but do not correlate with prognosis, which can be grave. Large areas of necrosis are seen histologically. Favorable responses to dapsone, as well as to replacement therapy with allogeneic α_1-antitrypsin, have been described. Pancreatic panniculitis, already discussed, comes under this heading.

Panniculitis associated with connective tissue disease – lupus profundus and morphea profunda. Lupus profundus is a rare variant of cutaneous lupus erythematosus (LE). Multiple, nontender nodules usually involve the face, upper arms, or buttocks. The nodules ulcerate and eventually leave irregular depressions. Characteristic histological changes of LE should be looked for in the dermis and epidermis. In morphea profunda, as in LE, a search should be made for histological evidence of scleroderma in the dermis. In the panniculus, a patchy lymphocytic infiltrate, often with plasma cells and eosinophils, orients towards the septae.

Infectious panniculitis. Adipose tissue is highly susceptible to infection in immunocompromised patients, in whom fungal (in particular *Aspergillus fumigatus*) rather than bacterial infections are more common. The infection may be percutaneous or, more commonly, systemic. Clinically these lesions are hard to diagnose, and culture is required.

Panniculitis associated with granulomatous diseases – sarcoidosis, granuloma annulare (**Fig. 2.9**), and necrobiosis lipoidica diabeticorum (**Fig. 2.10**). The latter two have characteristic clinical and histological features – the association with diabetes mellitus is much stronger for necrobiosis lipoidica than for granuloma annulare. Granuloma annulare usually resolves spontaneously within a couple of years, but necrobiosis lipoidica is difficult to treat, its course being unaffected by good diabetic control. Although potent topical steroid preparations have been used to treat both conditions, they should be avoided in necrobiosis lipoidica as they increase the risk of ulceration in an already thinned epidermis. Erythema nodosum with bihilar lymphadenopathy is characteristic of this form of sarcoidosis.

Panniculitis associated with thrombophlebitis. Inflammation of the veins in this condition may 'spill over' into the subcutaneous fat.

Others. It may not be possible to make a firm diagnosis on clinical or histological grounds, but the temptation to 'push' the diagnosis into one of the above categories should be resisted. Finally, it is worth mentioning that lymphomatous or leukemic infiltrates occasionally present with deep violaceous nodules when malignant cells invade the subcutaneous tissue.

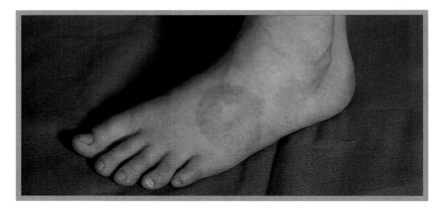

↑ Fig. 2.9
Granuloma annulare: the papular margins of this annular condition are distinctive. Lesions are pink in the early stages and then become more purple.

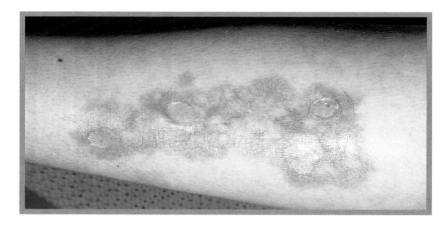

↑ Fig. 2.10
Necrobiosis lipoidica: thinning (atrophy) of the skin is striking, as are the yellow, brown, and pink discolourations and the numerous telangiectatic vessels.

3 | A traveller with diarrhoea

Case History

A 48-year-old woman was admitted to the infectious diseases unit with a 3-week history of persistent diarrhoea, which had begun while on a holiday in Mauritius. Ciproxin and metronidazole had been started a week before, but since then she had developed red eyes and painful red lesions on her arms, and complained of general malaise.

On admission she had a pyrexia, bilateral conjunctivitis, and discrete, red, tumid plaques on her neck (**Fig. 3.1**), hands, and arms (**Fig. 3.2**). A large apthous ulcer could be seen on her hard palate.

Results of investigations are shown in **Fig. 3.3**.

Sigmoidoscopy showed an inflamed rectal mucosa with contact bleeding. The histological changes of the rectal biopsy and the skin biopsy are shown in **Fig. 3.4** and **Figs 3.5a** and **b**, respectively.

Questions

1. **What is the diagnosis of the skin condition?**
2. **What is the bowel problem?**
3. **Are the skin and bowel conditions linked?**
4. **What other conditions can be associated with this skin disease?**

→ Fig. 3.1
These oedematous plaques are infiltrated with mature neutrophils.

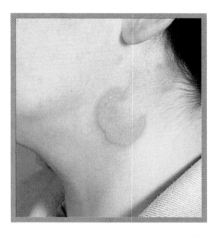

A traveller with diarrhoea

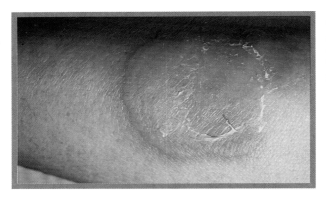

← **Fig. 3.2**
A tumid plaque
on the arm,
typical of this
condition.

Investigations	
FBC:	Hb 10.7g/dl
	(MCV 87.2, MCH 27.4)
WCC:	13.5×10^9/l (mainly neutrophils)
Platelets:	Normal
ESR:	80mm/h
CXR:	Normal
Stool cultures (×3):	No ova or parasites
Complement fixation tests for Chlamydia, Coxiella, and Mycoplasma	Negative

← **Fig. 3.3**
Table of
investigations.

→ Fig. 3.4
Granulomatous inflammation in the rectal mucosa.

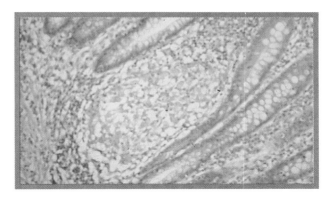

→ Fig. 3.5
(a) Skin biopsy revealing a superficial perivascular and interstitial infiltrate of neutrophils in a dermis that is grossly oedematous and showing incipient sub-epidermal vesiculation.
(b) Swollen endothelial cells and nuclear 'dust' of neutrophil origin are prominent. Fibrin is not seen in the vessel wall, therefore this is not a true vasculitis.

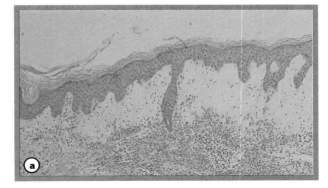

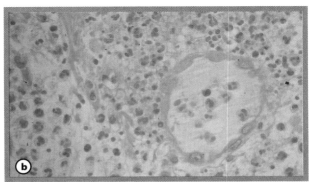

Answers

1. Sweet's syndrome (acute febrile neutrophilic dermatosis). This was described first, in 1964, by Robert Sweet. Its four cardinal features are fever, leukocytosis, tender red plaques, and a characteristic histology featuring an intense neutrophil infiltrate in the papillary dermis (without a true vasculitis). Cutaneous lesions are usually tender, bright to dusky red, raised papules or plaques, which heal with pigmentation. The plaques may be oval, round, or arcuate (**Fig. 3.6**), are sometimes vesicular (**Fig. 3.7**) or pustular, and most commonly affect the face or distal limbs.

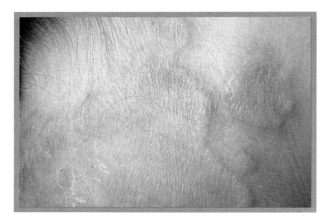

←**Fig. 3.6**
An arcuate lesion of Sweet's syndrome.

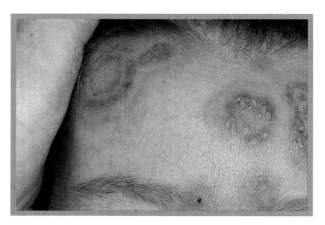

←**Fig. 3.7**
Annular erythematous plaques studded with closely set pseudovesicular papules.

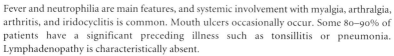

Fever and neutrophilia are main features, and systemic involvement with myalgia, arthralgia, arthritis, and iridocyclitis is common. Mouth ulcers occasionally occur. Some 80–90% of patients have a significant preceding illness such as tonsillitis or pneumonia. Lymphadenopathy is characteristically absent.

The ESR is invariably raised, and a neutrophil leukocytosis is common (60–80%). Liver function may be mildly deranged. Antineutrophil cytoplasmic antibody (ANCA, **Fig. 3.8**) was positive in all cases in one study of eight patients, but specific immunological abnormalities are not generally recognised.

The histology is characteristic and shows a patchy perivascular or dense band-like infiltrate in the upper and mid dermis. A variable admixture of lymphocytes and neutrophils are present, and the upper dermis may be markedly oedematous.

Other conditions to consider clinically include erythema multiforme, characterised by 'iris' and 'target' lesions, and urticaria, typified by evanescent, itchy, widespread lesions.

This condition responds dramatically to treatment with systemic corticosteroids, but anti-inflammatory agents such as aspirin and indomethacin, topical steroids, and potassium iodide have also been used with some success. The mechanism by which iodides act is unknown, but one possibility is that heparin release, brought about by iodide induced mast cell degranulation, inhibits delayed hypersensitivity.

2. Crohn's disease. Interestingly, this lady also had a yersinia infection (*Yersinia enterocolitica* serotype 03, titre 1:320), which has been reported in one previous case of Sweet's syndrome.

3. Crohn's disease is recognised to occur in association with Sweet's syndrome, as well as with other skin conditions:

→ Fig. 3.8
Immunofluorescence staining with classic antineutrophil cytoplasmic antibody (c-ANCA). There are several variants of this antibody: perinuclear ANCA (p-ANCA), a Henoch–Schönlein type IgA-ANCA, and a Goodpasture type IgM-ANCA.

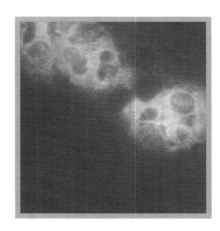

- Specific lesions – fissures, fistulas (**Fig. 3.9**), and metastatic Crohn's disease.
- Reactive lesions – erythema nodosum, pyoderma gangrenosum, apthous ulcers, necrotising vasculitis, Sweet's syndrome, and epidermolysis bullosa acquisita.
- Cutaneous manifestations secondary to complications:

(a) Malabsorption – acrodermatitis enteropathica, scurvy, purpura, pellagra, stomatitis/gingivitis.

(b) Secondary to treatment – drug eruptions, peristomal allergic/irritant dermatitis.

4. Sweet's syndrome can be associated with a range of other systemic diseases (in up to 50% of cases). Most important are the myeloproliferative disorders, including leukaemia, myeloma, lymphoma, and myelodysplasia. As discussed in Case 19, atypical forms of pyoderma gangrenosum and Sweet's syndrome have been reported with various forms of leukaemia, and may even occur simultaneously. Other conditions associated with Sweet's syndrome include ulcerative colitis, Crohn's disease, rheumatoid arthritis, Behçet's syndrome, and Sjögren's syndrome. Carcinoma of the testis, prostate, ovary, and vagina, in addition to metastatic adenocarcinoma, have also been reported in association with Sweet's syndrome. Nearly 10% of patients with Sweet's syndrome will have leukaemia, so a careful hematological evaluation and follow up are recommended.

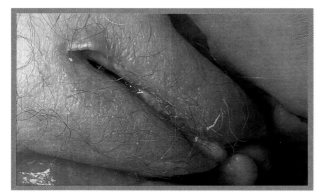

← Fig. 3.9
Fissures and fistulas are the commonest cutaneous manifestation of Crohn's disease. The perineum, especially the perianal region, is a site of predilection.

4 A man with a grey face

Case History

A 50-year-old man was referred to the clinic with gradually worsening pigmentation of his facial skin. He had been on minocycline, 100mg daily, for 10 years for a facial rash, but was otherwise well. On examination, the patient had slate-grey pigmentation of the forehead (**Fig. 4.1**), cheeks, and sclera (**Fig. 4.2**), but none in the mouth or trunk (**Fig. 4.3**).

→ Fig. 4.1
Severe greyish discolouration, most marked on the forehead.

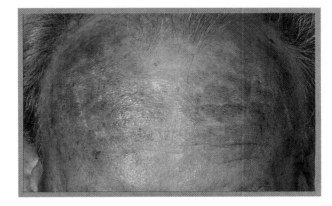

→ Fig. 4.2
Some pigmentation was also visible on the sclera.

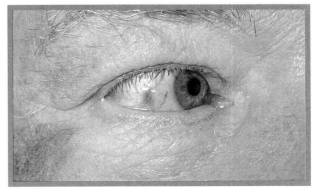

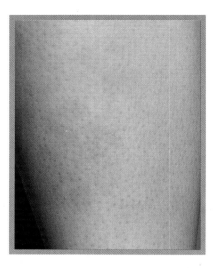

← Fig. 4.3
On the legs, a more bluish colour
could be seen.

Questions

1. What has caused the pigmentation?
2. What might produce a similar appearance, but occurs unilaterally?
3. What was the facial rash for which the patient was being treated?
4. How should this be treated?
5. What is the commonest cause of facial pigmentation in a woman?

Answers

1.   The pigmentation was due to minocycline. Some 2% of patients treated with this drug are so affected, usually those treated long term with high cumulative doses. Considered by some to be more effective than tetracycline and erythromycin, minocycline is often given for long periods to patients with acne. Minocycline-induced hyperpigmentation was first noted in the late 1970s and occurs in three forms. The first is characterised by dark, well defined, blue–black macules localised to depressed acne scars or the sites of inflammation. Hyperpigmented macules, or a diffuse hyperpigmentation away from sites of inflammation are typical of the second type, which is most common on the lower legs and sun-exposed areas (see **Fig. 4.3**). A third form, the 'muddy skin syndrome', is a diffuse dark, brown–grey discolouration, which may be generalised but most obvious on sun-exposed sites.

Tissue staining of organs other than the skin (sclera, thyroid, bone, and teeth) occurs also after long-term administration of minocycline. The pigment found in areas of previous inflammation is haemosiderin or a closely related iron-containing substance, whereas the skin in generalised minocycline hyperpigmentation contains excess melanin. The abnormal pigment in the 'muddy skin syndrome' may be a metabolic derivative of minocycline.

2. Confluent blue to brown macules in the distribution of the trigeminal nerve might suggest the nevus of Ota, a benign melanocytosis. Like minocycline-induced pigmentation, it frequently involves the sclera, cornea, or even the retina, but is unilateral. The condition is most common in young patients and persists. Treatment with recently available lasers may be effective. There is a small risk of malignant transformation of the retina, and patients should be assessed regularly by an ophthalmologist.

3. The minocycline was prescribed for rosacea. This disease is common, affecting 1 in 10 females between the ages of 35 and 50; prevalence is much less common for males. At first, the attacks of intense flushing – precipitated by alcohol, sunlight, drinks containing caffeine, hot or spicy foods, and changes in temperature – resolve rapidly. Later, the flushing episodes become more prolonged and the skin becomes red and telangectatic. Papules and pustules (**Figs 4.4** and **4.5**) develop. In severe rosacea, typically in men, the nose enlarges, reddens, and becomes rugose (known in Shakespearean times as 'grog blossom') (**Fig. 4.6**). Rosacea may also be associated with blepharitis and keratitis. Other conditions for which it may be mistaken include systemic lupus erythematosus, seborrhoeic dermatitis (although this is usually scaly and affects nasal folds), and contact dermatitis.

4. Rosacea is often misdiagnosed as acne vulgaris, which explains the serendipitous finding that tetracyclines are helpful. However, topical treatment should be tried first as it avoids the side effects of systemic antibiotic therapy. Useful information leaflets on triggering factors are now available. Moisturisers can help reduce the sensation of burning, but if this is unusually severe, hydrocortisone cream can be used for a short time. More potent topical steroids, and in particular fluorinated steroids, should be avoided as they may worsen the condition or induce a perioral dermatitis. Topical metronidazole is available as a water-based gel, but it

→ Fig. 4.4
Typical rosacea: the area of fixed erythema and telangiectasia on the cheeks continues to develop a series of red papules and pustules.

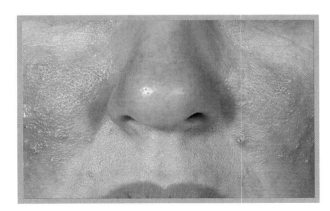

contains propylene glycol, a preservative that may irritate. Topical clindamycin (1% alcoholic solution or creamy lotion) is a suitable alternative, although is not yet licensed as a treatment for rosacea.

If topical treatment fails, systemic antibiotics should be started. These are particularly effective against the pustules, although less so for flushing. The reversal of erythema may reveal telangiectasia. This is known as the PERT phenomenon or posterythema revealed telangiectasia – patients should be warned about it. Oxytetracycline is the drug of first choice for rosacea, usually taken at the dose of 250mg four times daily, reducing after 2–3 months if a good response is achieved. However, although minocycline is expensive, it is popular with the patients and general practitioners as a once-daily medication.

5. Melasma is a common, acquired hypermelanosis in which brown macules appear symetrically and patches develop on sun-exposed areas. Females are predominantly affected and men make up only 10% of cases (**Fig. 4.7**). Predisposing factors include UV exposure, pregnancy, hormonal therapy, cosmetics, and phototoxic drugs. Based on Wood's light examination, melasma can be divided into three types. The epidermal variety has an increase in melanin throughout the epidermis, and the pigmentation is intensified by Wood's light. In dermal melasma, the pigmentation is not made more obvious by Wood's light. Both epidermal and dermal pigmentation is present in the mixed variety.

The treatment of melasma is unsatisfactory. Broad-spectrum sunscreens should be used regularly. Hydroquinone, which is available in some over-the-counter preparations, remains the most effective agent, but may produce ochronosis or even a confetti-like hypopigmentation, which is less acceptable than the melasma. Azelaic acid and laser therapy have also been used with some success.

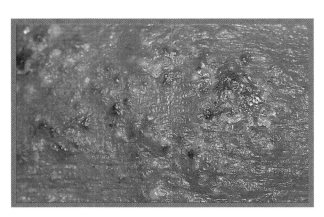

← Fig. 4.5
A close-up view of the papules and pustules of a more severe example of rosacea.

→ Fig. 4.6
The thickened red nose of rhinophyma is often associated with rosacea.

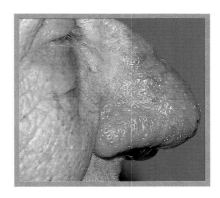

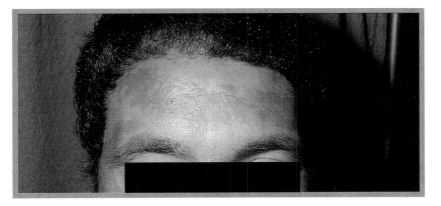

↑ Fig. 4.7
Remember that melasma can occur, although uncommonly, in men.

5 | A rash stroke

Case History

This 46-year-old woman had first attended our clinic 25 years ago, with red, scaly plaques on her forehead, nose, and cheeks (**Fig. 5.1**). A range of investigations, including FBC, ESR, full biochemical screen, urinalysis, serum immunoglobulins, complement profile, and antinuclear factor (ANF), had all been normal or negative, and a skin biopsy was also performed. Over the next 8 years, her skin disease was well controlled by potent topical corticosteroids and intermittent courses of a systemic agent. During the next 14 years, the immunological and hematological abnormalities detailed in **Fig. 5.2** were detected.

She then developed right lower lobe pneumonia and emphysema (**Fig. 5.3**), but no organism could be isolated from sputum, pleural aspirate, or blood cultures, and the pneumoccal antigen titre was negative. Nevertheless, this episode responded to intravenous antibiotics.

Six years ago, this eruption appeared on her thighs (**Fig. 5.4**) and periungal erythema was noted (**Fig. 5.5**). Three years ago, she developed sensory loss over the extensor surface of the left arm and weakness of the extensors and flexors of the left wrist. Lumbar puncture, CT scan, and visual evoked responses gave no evidence of multiple sclerosis. She then developed expressive and receptive dysphasia, and a repeat CT scan showed probable cerebral infarction (**Fig. 5.6**). At that time, an elevated titre of a specific antibody was detected, and treatment was started with azathioprine and warfarin. Nifedipine was required within a few months for hypertension.

→ **Fig. 5.1**
Typical, well-defined, erythematous, scaly plaques. Closer inspection will reveal keratotic plugs in the openings of hair follicles.

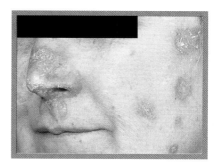

← Fig. 5.2
Table of investigations.

Test result	No. of years after initial presentation
ANF positive	8
Thrombocytopenia	12
Anti-DNA titre 65iu/l	14

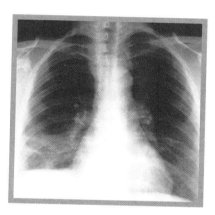

← Fig. 5.3
There is increased density over the right lower zone with loss of definition of the hemidiaphragm, indicating some consolidation and collapse of the right lower lobe. There is also a small pleural effusion.

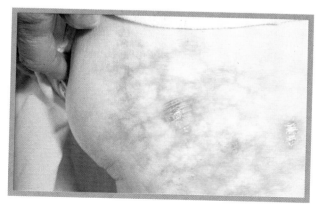

← Fig. 5.4
The eruption that appeared on the patient's thighs (see answer to question 1).

A rash stroke

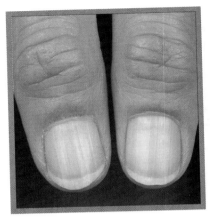

↑ Fig. 5.5
Redness and telangiectasia of the proximal nail folds. Similar changes may occur in dermatomyositis (see Fig. 1.5) and systemic sclerosis.

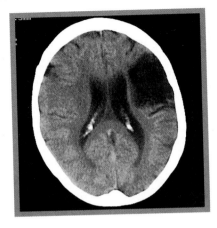

↑ Fig. 5.6
This CT scan of the brain shows an obvious left-sided infarct.

Questions

1. What are the skin changes shown in Fig. 5.4? What can cause them?
2. What disease does this patient have, and what is the differential diagnosis?
3. What are the three main cutaneous subtypes of this condition?
4. What drug was prescribed for her skin disease? Are other treatment options available?
5. Which specific antibody was elevated, and what does this imply?

Answers

1. This is livedo reticularis. The purplish network of lines is due to stagnation of blood in capillaries lying at the boundaries between areas of skin supplied by individual arterioles. The pattern is similar to that seen in the transient physiological mottling (cutis marmorata) shown by some children after exposure to cold, and to erythema *ab igne*.

As well as this patient's condition (see later), important underlying causes of livedo reticularis include polyarteritis nodosa, cryoglobinemia, and thrombocytopenia.

2. This patient had the characteristic features of discoid lupus erythematosus (LE). The face is most commonly affected, but the scalp, nose, ears, limbs, and trunk can also be involved. Lesions of discoid LE resolve with hyperpigmentation or hypopigmentation, commonly leaving atrophy and telangiectasia. It can also cause scarring alopecia.

Other conditions that can be confused with discoid LE include:

Discoid eczema. This is easily ruled out by histology and immunofluorescence. It is usually itchy, responds rapidly to topical corticosteroids, and does not scar.

Acne/rosacea. Approximately 8% of patients with discoid LE have a rosacea-like pattern with red papules on the central face and chin, but the pustules, so typical of true rosacea, are not found.

Polymorphic light eruption. This photosensitive eruption typically affects young females on sun-exposed sites. In many patients it appears on the first sunny day of spring, although in some it is provoked only by exceptionally hot weather. The typical features are coloured or erythematous papules, coalescing to form plaques. All patients show tachyphylaxis, in that the rash gradually improves with repeated sun exposure.

Lupus vulgaris. This usually occurs at an earlier age, and has characteristic 'apple jelly nodules'.

3. The criteria for the diagnosis of systemic LE (SLE) were established by the American Rheumatism Association (ARA) in 1982. Histopathologically, the cutaneous manifestations of SLE cannot be distinguished from discoid LE, which is characterised by moderately dense lymphocytic infiltrates around venules of the superficial and deep plexuses, with vacuolar alteration and a focal thinning of the epidermis. IgG, IgA, IgM, and complement are found at the dermo-epidermal junction of involved skin in about 80% of patients (**Fig. 5.7**). In contrast, immunoreactants are found in uninvolved skin in SLE.

The cutaneous manifestations of SLE may include leukocytoclastic vasculitis, blisters, deep ulcers above the medial malleoli, calcinosis cutis, and diffuse alopecia. The well-known malar rash is usually transient (**Fig. 5.8**). Discoid lesions are uncommon in SLE, and only some 6% of patients with discoid LE have systemic involvement. Most patients with discoid LE, therefore, have a good prognosis despite the sometimes disfiguring and scarring lesions.

The third distinct subset of LE, first described in 1979, is subacute cutaneous LE (SCLE). characteristic of this subtype are annular or polycyclic lesions (**Fig. 5.9**) or a papulosquamous rash, predominantly of the upper trunk. Some 50% of patients with SCLE fulfill the ARA criteria for the diagnosis of SLE, and the associated systemic disease usually involves the musculoskeletal system. Photosensitivity is a prominent feature, but renal or CNS involvement is rare.

→ Fig. 5.7
Immunohistology of involved skin in a patient with discoid lupus erythematosus, showing IgG deposition at the dermoepidermal junction.

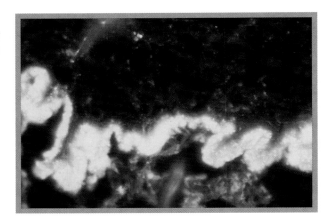

→ Fig. 5.8
The 'butterfly' rash of systemic lupus erythematosus.

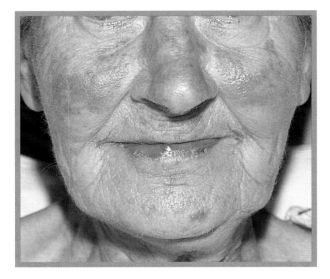

4. The patient was given hydoxychloroquine. If topical measures, such as the regular use of sunscreens and application of potent steroids, fail to control discoid LE, an oral antimalarial is the drug of first choice. Hydroxychloroquine, up to 800mg twice daily, is preferred to chloroquine sulfate, which is cheaper but has greater side effects. The serious side effects of these antimalarials include corneal deposition and retinopathy. They can be avoided by asking patients regularly about visual symptoms, especially photophobia, and by examining the fundus. Self-testing for visual field abnormalities (using an Amsler chart – **Fig. 5.10**). Antimalarials should be stopped during the winter to minimise cumulative toxicity. Prednisolone, up to 15mg daily, may be tried if the above measures are unsuccessful. Clofazamine, gold, dapsone, etretinate, cyclosporin A, and cyclophosphamide are effective in discoid LE, but their side effects put them on the 'reserve' list.

5. The anticardiolipin antibody was elevated. The presence of antiphospholipid antibodies, measured as anticardiolipin antibodies or as the similar lupus anticoagulant, is associated with an increased risk of venous and arterial thromboses, thrombocytopenia, pulmonary hypertension, and recurrent spontaneous abortion. The term antiphospholipid syndrome covers this combination of clinical and serological features. Livedo reticularis or vasculitis, thrombophlebitis, cutaneous infarcts, and discoid LE are the main cutaneous changes. The most sensitive test for antiphospholipid antibodies is the anticardiolipin antibody test, in which ELISA or solid-phase radioimmunoassay techniques are used to demonstrate antibody binding to solid plates coated with cardiolipin or other negatively charged phospholipids. Approximately 15% of patients with discoid LE, and 25% of those with SLE, are anticardiolipin positive. The complications depend on specificity, isotype, and level. Corticosteroid therapy lowers anticardiolipin antibody titres but may not lower the risk of thrombosis, and so is probably justified only in patients with continuing episodes of thrombosis despite adequate anticoagulation. Subcutaneous heparin and antiplatelet agents, alone or in combination, have also been used as prophylactic measures.

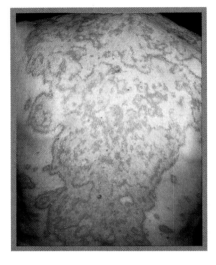

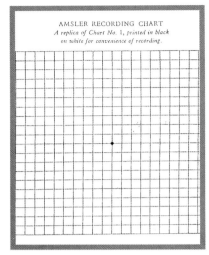

AMSLER RECORDING CHART
A replica of Chart No. 1, printed in black on white for convenience of recording.

↑ Fig. 5.9
Note the erythematous polycylic lesions, in a characteristic distribution over the back and shoulders.

↑ Fig. 5.10
An Amsler chart: patients should hold the chart at reading distance and then cover one eye at a time while focusing on the center point. If they cannot see the grid in all quadrants, this should be reported to the doctor.

6 | Pain and proteinuria

Case History

A 22-year-old man presented with an extensive rash on the legs, buttocks, and forearms, subsequent to a sore throat. He also complained of pain and swelling in his ankles and elbows. He denied any recent medication or travel abroad.

On examination, the patient had a palpable rash on the sites listed above (**Figs 6.1** and **6.2**), with marked swelling and tenderness over both ankles. A wide range of investigations (**Fig. 6.3**), including a skin biopsy (**Fig. 6.4**), were undertaken.

The rash worsened over the next week, but then settled on a reducing course of prednisolone. During the next 2 years, the patient had several recurrences of the rash on dependent sites, often after a sore throat. These episodes were managed conservatively until he developed microscopic hematuria and proteinuria, and then showed significant renal impairment (**Fig. 6.5**). A repeat punch skin biopsy for direct immunofluorescence showed the deposition of a specific immunoglobulin around dermal blood vessels (**Fig. 6.6**). The patient was referred for renal biopsy (**Fig. 6.7**).

→ Fig. 6.1
Painful purpura, most severe on the lower legs, where some lesions are becoming necrotic.

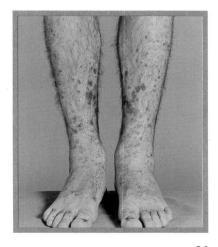

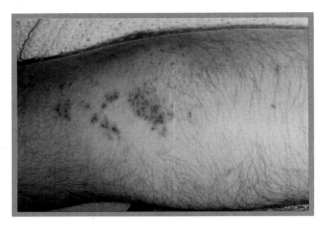

← Fig. 6.2
The left elbow joint is swollen and there is overlying purpura.

Investigations	
FBC, ESR, biochemical profile, and urinalysis:	Normal
Antistreptolysin-O titer:	200u/ml
Viral screen, including hepatitis screen:	Negative
Serum IgA:	5.5g/l (normal=0.5–4.0g/l)
Other immunoglobulins:	Normal
ANA:	Negative
Complement profile:	Normal
Cryoglobulins and cold aggulutinins:	Negative

← Fig. 6.3
Table of investigations.

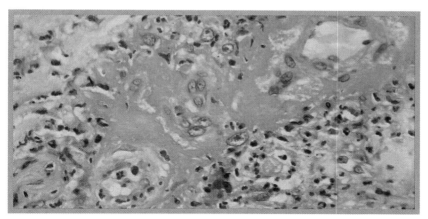

↑ Fig. 6.4

This skin biopsy shows a leukocytoclastic vasculitis (synonymous with 'allergic' or 'necrotizing' vasculitis) which is characterized by fibrin within the walls of small dermal venules, and thrombi within their lumina, in association with an inflammatory infiltrate. The infiltrate is composed mainly of neutrophils, and there is also nuclear debris (dust) and extravasated red blood cells.

→ Fig. 6.5
Results of renal investigations.

Renal Investigations	
Urinalysis: (during an active phase)	Protein ++, blood ++
Urine casts:	None seen microscopically
24-h creatinine clearance:	70ml/min (>l00ml/min)
24-h urinary protein:	<0.3g/24h

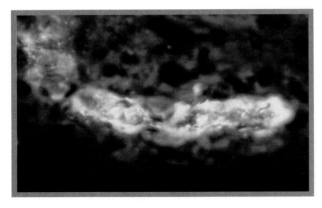

← Fig. 6.6
Direct immuno-
fluorescence
staining of a skin
biopsy shows IgA
deposition
around dermal
blood vessels.

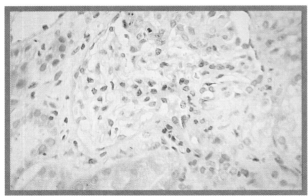

← Fig. 6.7
Renal biopsy
shows focal and
sclerosing
mesangio-
proliferative
glomerulo-
nephritis.

Questions

1. What is the diagnosis for this patient?
2. Does the skin immunohistology allow you to make a firm diagnosis?
3. How should the condition be managed and what is the patient's
   overall prognosis?

Answers

1. Leukocytoclastic (allergic) vasculitis. All small vessel vasculitides (e.g. leukocytoclastic vasculitis, septic vasculitis, livedo vasculitis) may be associated with localized bleeding into the skin (purpura), but inflammatory skin diseases (e.g. erythema multiforme) and fixed drug eruptions can also cause this. Noninflammatory processes, such as trauma to sun-damaged skin (solar purpura – **Fig. 6.8**) and coagulation disorders, should also be considered.

To divide vasculitis into cutaneous and systemic types is often not possible without full and repeated investigations. A detailed history may provide clues to possible triggers such as infections, drugs, foods, connective tissue disease, diabetes, chronic respiratory or bowel disease, or malignancy. Recurrent throat infections seemed to have been the triggering factor in this case, although negative throat swabs and the ASO titre did not support this idea.

Purpura should not be confused with petechiae, which result from a capillaritis. Inflammation of capillaries is the basic pathological process in a group of conditions called the pigmented purpuric dermatoses (**Fig. 6.9**). These usually affect the lower legs and feet of middle-aged men and are thought to be caused, in part, by venous insufficiency. The dermatoses are invariably asymptomatic, and have no recognized treatment.

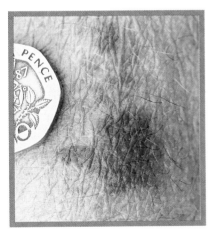

↑ Fig. 6.8
Solar purpura on the arm of an Australian patient.

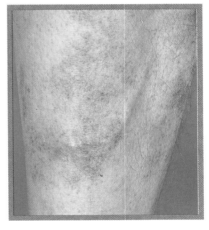

↑ Fig. 6.9
Pinhead-sized petechiae and red-brown pigmentation, due to the leakage of red blood cells and deposition of haemosiderin in the surrounding tissue.

2. Yes and no. IgG, IgM, IgA, and complement may be deposited around blood vessels in the early stages of immune-complex-mediated leukocytoclastic vasculitis, but the deposition of IgA alone is the hallmark of Henoch–Schönlein purpura (HSP). Some regard a raised serum level of IgA, or its deposition in the skin, as diagnostic of HSP. However, HSP is distinctive clinically – as an urticarial/purpuric rash, mainly on the lower legs and buttocks, with arthritis, or gastrointestinal symptoms, or both. Two-thirds of affected individuals have abdominal symptoms such as colic, vomiting, or diarrhoea, often accompanied by hematemesis or rectal bleeding. Polyarthritis occurs in most cases. HSP is most common in childhood, and nephritis is an important complication. IgA and C3 may be been found on immunofluorescence of renal biopsy specimens, which show focal proliferative glomerulonephritis.

3. In the absence of renal involvement, continuous – or even intermittent – oral steroid therapy is not indicated. Neither the course of the disease nor the incidence of renal involvement will be altered by steroids. Bed rest is the best therapy. Urinalysis should be carried out weekly during the acute phase, at the end of an attack, and at 1–3 months after an attack has subsided. Episodes usually last 3–6 weeks, but recurrences are seen in up to 50% of patients and may continue for several years. The prognosis depends on the degree and severity of renal involvement. Some 25% of patients with renal involvement later develop chronic nephritis. The prognosis is not influenced by the age at onset, the relapse rate, or the presence of streptococcal infection.

7 | Flat and shiny

Case History

A 35-year-old man developed an itchy rash which started on his wrists (**Fig. 7.1**) and extended to involve his trunk. Linear lesions developed on traumatized areas (**Fig. 7.2**), and there were also changes in his mouth (**Fig. 7.3**) and subtle abnormalities of his nails (**Fig. 7.4**). He was on no medication.

→ Fig. 7.1
These polygonal, shiny papules are characteristic of this condition, as is involvement of the flexor side of the wrist.

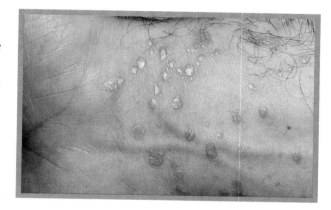

→ Fig. 7.2
Like psoriasis and sarcoidosis, this skin disease demonstrates the Köebner phenomenon (i.e. it appears at sites of trauma).

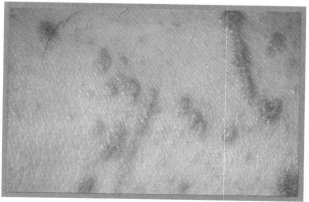

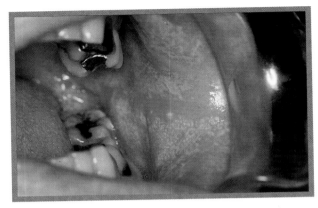

Flat and shiny

← **Fig. 7.3**
These lacy, white reticulate changes are typical of the condition.

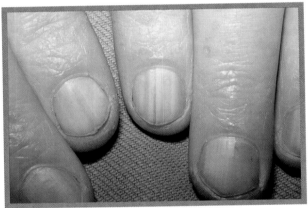

← **Fig. 7.4**
Thinning and longitudinal ridging are characteristic early nail changes.

Questions

1. What is the diagnosis?
2. Can other appendygeal structures be involved?
3. What are the associated liver abnormalities?
4. What are the main histological features of this skin disease?
5. What is the differential diagnosis?
6. How would you treat this patient?

Answers

1. This is lichen planus (LP), which is characterized by violaceous flat topped papules, often mainly on flexor surfaces, and by white reticulate lesions on the mucous membranes and genitalia.

The aetiology of LP is unknown. Favored hypotheses include a viral cause, immunological abnormalities (a similar rash can be seen in graft-versus-host disease), neurological changes, and emotional stress.

Lesions vary greatly in size, but usually have a distinctive, shiny, flat-topped appearance with a whitish lacy network over the surface (Wickham's striae – **Fig. 7.5**). Linear lesions often appear along scratch marks (Köebner phenomenon). Several variants of LP are recognized, including hypertrophic LP (**Fig. 7.6**) and bullous LP (acute LP – **Fig. 7.7**).

→ Fig. 7.5
Wickham's striae are due to areas of compact orthokeratosis lying above the zones of hypergranulosis.

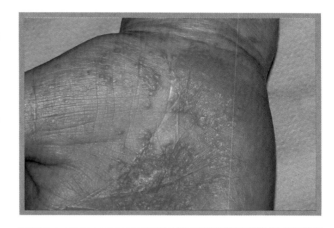

→ Fig. 7.6
Hypertrophic lichen planus may be a reaction to repeated rubbing – note the excoriations here.

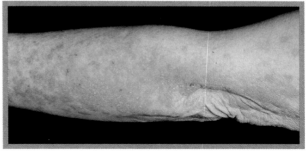

Flat and shiny

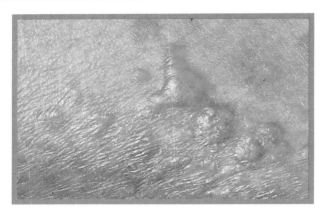

← Fig. 7.7
The presence of bullae implies that the lichen planus is acute.

Mucous membrane lesions are common (seen in 30–70% of patients) and can occur without any lesions on the skin. The reticulate white streaks on the buccal mucosa are quite distinctive; and those on the tongue are usually fixed, white, and sometimes slightly depressed plaques. The mouth is most often involved, but lesions may be found around the anus or on the genitalia. Itching is usual, but occasionally lesions are asymptomatic. Mouth lesions can sting or hurt, and ulcerated ones are especially painful. LP is confined to the mouth, or has only minimal skin involvement, in 15% of cases.

2.   The nails are involved in about 10% of patients, most frequently in severe generalized LP. The commonest change is a slight thinning of the nail plate as it emerges from under the cuticle, with exaggeration of the normal longitudinal lines and a transverse linear depression of the nail plate. Onycholysis, subungal hyperkeratosis, and nail shedding (**Fig. 7.8**) also occur, and pterygium formation is characteristic. Rarely, a nail may be completely destroyed. LP

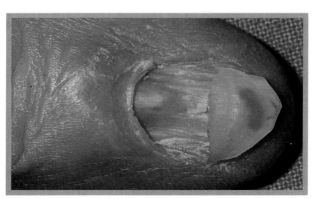

← Fig. 7.8
This nail has become thinned proximally and the distal part is about to separate off.

can also cause alopecia, although this is rare. The inflammatory infiltrate extends deeply around hair follicles, and ultimately destroys them by scarring. Typically this creates small areas of atrophic scarring alopecia on the scalp.

3. The reported prevalence of liver disease in patients with LP ranges from 0.1 to 35%. Chronic active hepatitis of unknown cause is the most common association, but primary biliary cirrhosis has also occasionally been linked with LP. In most of these cases, the diagnosis was made by a single determination of serum aminotransferase activity. Recent studies suggest that when chronic liver disease is associated with LP, hepatitis C virus (HCV) is its cause (**Fig. 7.9**). The reported prevalence of HCV in LP varies from 4 to 38%, but a causal relationship between HCV and LP remains to be established.

4. The characteristic histological features of LP are hyperkeratosis, wedge-shaped zones of hypergranulosis (**Fig. 7.10**), and irregular epidermal hyperplasia (acanthosis) resulting in a 'saw tooth' appearance of the epidermis. The upper dermis contains a band-like infiltrate of lymphocytes which obscures the dermo-epidermal junction, along which vacuoles and necrotic keratinocytes – referred to as colloid, cytoid, or Civatte bodies – are usually seen.

5. The main differential diagnosis is a lichenoid eruption caused by a drug. Many drugs can produce a lichenoid reaction pattern, but gold is probably the most common. Other offenders include thiazide diuretics, isoniazid, streptomycin, and methyldopa. Some, such as quinine or demeclocyline, require light exposure before an LP-like eruption occurs. Drug-induced lesions tend to be more psoriasiform than true LP, and, histologically, the infiltrate is sparser and colloid bodies are found more superficially in the epidermis.

6. Topical steroids, emollients, and antihistamines help mild to moderately severe LP. High potency topical steroids may be used at the start, but lower potency preparations are preferred, whenever possible, for maintenance. Oral corticosteroids are helpful in severe symptomatic disease, and a 2- to 8-week tapering course may lead to a complete clearance. However, there is a high rate of relapse. Hypertrophic lesions respond to potent topical steroids under occlusion, and to intralesional corticosteroid injections.

→ Fig. 7.9
Table of skin diseases associated with hepatitis C virus (HCV) infection.

Skin diseases associated with HCV infection
Porphyria cutanea tarda
Lichen planus
Cutaneous vasculitis
Polyarteritis nodosa
Erythema nodosum
Erythema multiforme
Prurigo
Urticaria

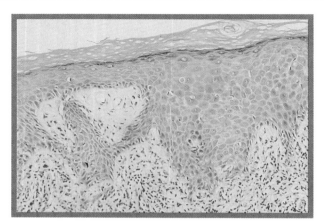

← Fig. 7.10
Wedge-shaped areas of hypergranulosis (thickening of the granular cell layer) are the most consistent finding at all stages and in every manifestation of lichen planus.

Symptomatic oral lesions can be treated with topical corticosteroids such as fluocinonide gel or triamcinolone in an oral adhesive base (Orabase); severe oral involvement may require a short reducing course of systemic steroids.

A number of other systemic agents have been used to treat LP, but with variable success. These include griseofulvin, systemic retinoids, and low-dose cyclophosphamide. Photochemotherapy (PUVA) may also help.

8 | Hark the herald!

Case History

A 25-year-old semiprofessional cyclist came to the emergency department with an itchy, widespread rash of acute onset. Four days before the rash had become widespread, he had noticed a large pink patch on one shoulder. The patient also complained of mild flu-like symptoms. He was on no current medication. On examination, his widespread eruption consisted of discrete, pink, oval lesions with a collarette of scales pointing centrally (**Fig. 8.1**). The distribution of the rash was also distinctive (**Fig. 8.2**).

A number of investigations were performed (**Fig. 8.3**). The patient was reassured and treated symptomatically.

→ Fig. 8.1
The characteristic rim of scaling is lying inside the edge of a lesion.

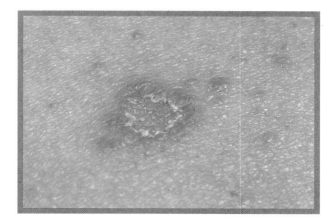

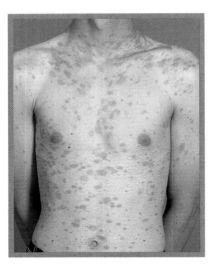

← Fig. 8.2
The characteristic lesions are most numerous in a T-shirt distribution.

← Fig. 8.3
Table of investigations.

Investigations

FBC: normal

Viral titres (both immediate and convalescent): normal

VDRL and TPHA: negative

Examination of a potassium hydroxide preparation of scrapings of a lesion for mycology: no evidence of fungal hyphae

Questions

1. What is the diagnosis for this patient?
2. What is the differential diagnosis?
3. Could any drug cause this reaction?

Answers

1. Pityriasis rosea. This common, acute, self-limiting rash usually affects children or young adults. A viral cause has been suspected – but not proven – because of the rapid onset, the seasonal variations in incidence, the rarity of recurrences, and sporadic reports of case clustering. Mild leukopenia with relative lymphocytosis may occur at the peak of the eruption, providing further evidence for a viral aetiology.

The clinical presentation is usually so characteristic that a history and physical examination are sufficient to make the diagnosis. Prodromal symptoms occasionally occur, and the first sign of the rash is the appearance of a 'herald patch' (**Fig. 8.4**), typically larger than the other lesions, which appear in crops 3–14 days later. Individual lesions are round or oval, erythematous papules and plaques with an inner collarette of scale. The rash occupies a 'T-shirt' distribution (i.e. it rarely extends beyond the mid upper arms or neck) and lesions tend to follow the lines of the dermatomes (**Figs 8.5** and **8.6**) and so may create a 'Christmas tree' pattern on the back. New lesions continue to appear over a few weeks, persist for few weeks, and then gradually resolve. 'Pityriasis', meaning 'bran-like', describes the fine scale seen in this condition (**Fig. 8.7**).

→ Fig. 8.4
The largest lesion, above the umbilicus, is a fading herald patch. At this stage, many other smaller lesions are beginning to appear.

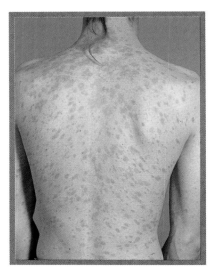

← Fig. 8.5
Individual lesions are oval, and their long axes tend to lie along dermatomal lines.

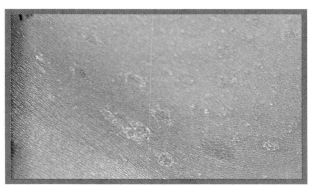

← Fig. 8.6
Scaly collarettes show up particularly well on pigmented skin. The long axes of the lesions again seem to lie along dermatomal lines.

→ Fig. 8.7
A reminder that
the word
'pityriasis' means
'bran-like'.

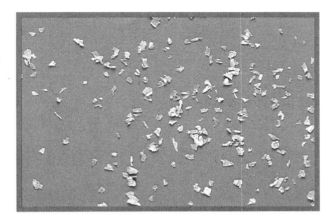

A biopsy is necessary only in atypical cases, and the histological features are suggestive rather than diagnostic. Patients should be reassured about the benign and self-limiting nature of the rash. Topical steroids and oral antihistamines are helpful for pruritus, which is occasionally severe.

2. The differential diagnosis of pityriasis rosea is wide and includes many papulosquamous rashes, for example:

Parapsoriasis (digitate dermatosis, see Case 22) – several subtypes of parapsoriasis exist, but the small-plaque type most resembles pityriasis rosea, with its oval patches or barely raised plaques, which tend to run horizontally, and parallel to each other. The chronicity of the condition and the lack of evolving and resolving lesions distinguish this condition from pityriasis rosacea.

Seborrhoeic dermatitis – this may be pityriasiform, but its lesions develop slowly, mainly in the upper central trunk and scalp. They are duller in colour and the scales are thicker and more greasy. The rash persists if untreated.

Secondary syphilis – although this is classically the great mimicker, the resemblance in this case is not close. It should be kept in mind, however, as the incidence of syphilis is increasing with the spread of HIV infection. Between 27 and 35% of HIV-positive patients have syphilis, but the serology may be negative and dark field microscopy is indicated if the diagnosis is suspected. HIV infection does not alter the course of syphilis. The rash of secondary syphilis has poorly defined lesions (**Fig. 8.8**), which typically also involve the palms and soles. It may be brown or red, and tends to be papular with a tightly adherent scale. Annular plaques on the mouth and nose are virtually diagnostic of secondary syphilis, and develop 6–12 weeks after the primary chancre, which itself lasts 4–6 weeks. Shin pain is a distinctive feature of syphilis and provides a useful diagnostic clue.

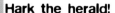

Guttate psoriasis – the lesions are usually papular and persistent, with silvery scales (**Fig. 8.9**). The onset of the eruption is often preceded by a streptococcal sore throat.

Tinea corporis – the herald patch of pityriasis rosea may be confused with ringworm, but the latter is more oedematous and may show marginal vesiculation. Microscopic examination of scrapings from the edge of the lesion will confirm the diagnosis of ringworm.

3. Several drugs can cause pityriasiform reactions: these include barbiturates, clonidine, captopril, metronidazole, and ketotifen. Such drug-induced eruptions tend to be more symptomatic, may become lichenoid, and are not associated with a typical herald patch.

← Fig. 8.8
A symmetric eruption with little scaling at this stage. Look for lesions on the palms and soles.

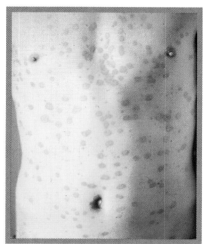

← Fig. 8.9
This patient's lesions started as guttate psoriasis, but have now evolved into small plaques.

9 | Right on target?

Case History

A 44-year-old man had first developed painful blisters and erosions on his lips and oral mucosa 29 years previously. He also had occasional erosions and vesiculopustular lesions on his forearms and hands. A number of investigations were performed at that stage (**Fig. 9.1**). Since then, he has suffered recurrent episodes of severe oral (**Fig. 9.2**) and nasal (**Fig. 9.3**) ulceration, invariably associated with lesions on the hands and forearms (**Fig. 9.4**).

He has also occasionally had herpes labialis, occurring about 1 week before the onset of recurrences of his rash, but specific tests have yielded a positive result on one occasion only, 5 years ago (**Fig. 9.5**). He is a chronic alcohol abuser, and has abused drugs in the past. He also received a course of antituberculous therapy 10 years ago, after acid-fast bacilli had been found in sputum samples.

→ Fig. 9.1
Table of initial investigations.

Investigations	
FBC:	Normal
Full biochemical screen:	Normal
ANA:	Negative
Serum immunoglobulins:	Normal
Complement profile:	Normal

→ Fig. 9.2
Ulceration and crusting of the lips.

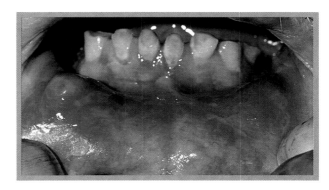

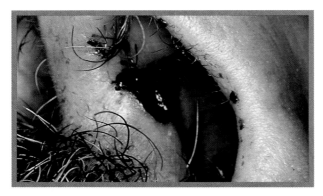

← Fig. 9.3
Haemorrhagic crusting inside the nasal rims.

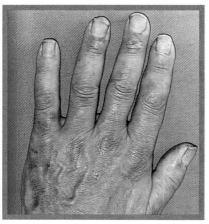 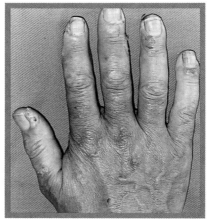

↑ Fig. 9.4
Erosions and crusting on the hands.

Questions

1. What is the diagnosis for this patient?
2. Which are the most common precipitating factors?
3. What other investigations could be used to confirm herpesvirus infection?
4. What complications can arise with the more severe form of this eruption?

Table of later
investigations.

Investigations	
Viral swabs:	Negative
HSV antibodies (immunoadherence hemagglutinin assay):	Repeatedly negative
HSV complement fixation test:	Positive on one occasion

Answers

1. Erythema multiforme (EM). This is an acute, self-limiting condition with distinctive skin lesions, with or without mucosal lesions. The concept of EM has become a little confused because physicians apply the name to various rashes and incorrectly use the term 'multiforme' to denote the presence at one time of different types of skin lesions. The fact that 'multiforme' was originally used to describe the evolution of individual skin lesions, is often forgotten.

Hebra described an acute, self-limiting, mild skin disease comprising symmetrically distributed skin lesions mainly on the extremities, with a tendency to recur, often at the same time of year. He also described the evolution of the skin lesions and their concentric colour changes (**Fig. 9.6**), which create the typical target lesions of EM.

As the lesions resolve, they become scaly, and although they do not produce scarring, postinflammatory pigmentation is usual. The morphology of the eruption in EM major is variable and often atypical – hence, the classic target lesions may not be seen. The more usual

Fig. 9.6
A typical target
lesion with a
peripheral rim of
erythema
surrounding a
pale center. The
bull's eye is
either
erythematous or
vesicular.

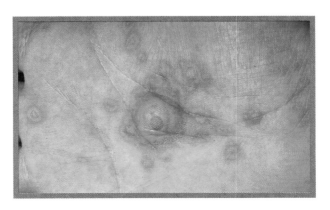

rash in this form of EM is maculopapular, with confluent areas of erythema, large bullae, large plaques, and a massive denudation of the epidermis like that seen in toxic epidermal necrolysis. Many of these features, described by Hebra in 1866, remain valid today, but it is now recognised that mucosal lesions occur in up to 60% of cases of EM minor.

Stevens–Johnson syndrome is a severe form of EM (**Figs 9.7** and **9.8**). The first two cases described by Stevens and Johnson were boys with acute febrile illnesses, associated with EM-like skin lesions and severe purulent conjunctivitis, which resulted in permanent visual impairment.

Management of our patient was with local treatment (tetracycline/steroid mouthwash preparations and topical steroids) and intermittent courses of systemic immunosuppressive agents, including prednisolone, azathioprine, and dapsone. Over the past 5 years, however, he has been maintained on low-dose acyclovir, which has reduced the frequency of his attacks.

2. Most of the precipitating factors of EM are either infectious agents or drugs, and the following are well documented.

(a) Herpes (HSV)-associated EM.

The proportion of herpes-associated cases in published series ranges from 15 to 60%. EM typically follows a HSV infection within 1–3 weeks, and in young adults. The EM, like the associated HSV lesions, frequently recurs, and both HSV type-1 and type-2 infections can act as triggers.

EM is thought to be a hypersensitivity phenomenon to the viral particles, which have occasionally been isolated from lesions. EM may also be associated with asymptomatic HSV carriage, and HSV DNA has recently been detected in involved epidermis. Low-dose oral acyclovir prevents recrudescent HSV infection in these patients. It has been speculated that most EM-minor attacks are herpes associated. Upper respiratory tract infections, sunlight, X-rays, tuberculosis, menses, and certain drugs can all reactivate the virus, and this explains the apparent association of EM with such a wide range of factors.

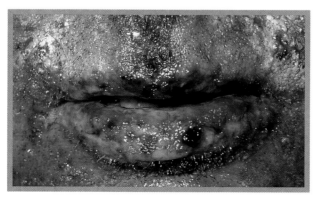

← Fig. 9.7
Gross mouth and lip ulceration in a patient with severe Stevens–Johnson syndrome.

→ Fig. 9.8
The same patient – who, sadly, died of septicemia – showing the extent of his skin involvement.

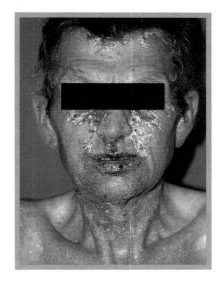

(b) Mycoplasma-associated EM.

A clear association between EM and infections with *Mycoplasma pneumoniae* has been documented over the last 30 years. This occurs typically in children and young adults, and usually follows infection with *M. pneumoniae* within days or weeks. In contrast to herpes-associated EM, such an illness is usually characterised by multiple lesions on mucosal surfaces and large skin blisters.

(c) Drug associated EM.

The best-documented association is with sulfonamides, particularly the long-acting ones. Sulfonamide-associated EM appears typically after 7–14 days of therapy, but may occur within hours. Sulfonamide EM is characterised by fever and prostration, and is usually an EM major. Large bullae, confluent erythema, or even a toxic erythema necrolysis-like picture, may be seen on the skin, and extensive, severe mucosal lesions are characteristic. Other well-documented precipitating drugs are phenylbutazone, diphenylhydantoin, and penicillin derivatives. Many of the drugs associated with EM major can cause other patterns of cutaneous hypersensitivity, such as urticaria, maculopapular drug eruptions, and fixed drug eruptions.

3. A Tzanck smear and a skin biopsy may confirm herpesvirus infection. In 1947, Tzanck reported that the cytological examination of smears obtained from vesicles caused by herpes simplex, herpes zoster, and varicella allowed a rapid diagnosis to be made based on the finding of pathognomonic giant cells. Mitotic nuclear division may result in the formation of a single large nucleus or multiple syncytial nuclei, which mould together in a jigsaw puzzle-like fashion. It is unusual to see these giant cells in very early lesions of infection by herpesvirus.

A skin biopsy (**Fig. 9.9**) is also useful in the diagnosis of mucocutaneous HSV infection and can establish the diagnosis of other cutaneous conditions that clinically mimic an HSV infection, such as vesicular eczematous dermatitis or a recurrent fixed drug eruption of the genitalia. Older vesicles caused by herpesvirus show epidermal necrosis and it may not be possible to identify multinucleated giant epithelial cells. A search for the ghost of these multinucleated acantholytic cells may then confirm the diagnosis.

4.   Typical EM minor is relatively benign, with no significant complications. EM major, in contrast, commonly leads to serious complications, with the eyes most frequently affected. Visual impairment can occur in the acute stage, due to keratitis, or later with conjunctival scarring. Permanent visual impairment follows in up to 10% of patients with ocular involvement. Involvement of the upper airways and pneumonia is seen in up to 30% of cases of EM major. It is not clear whether the associated pneumonia is a complication of airway involvement by EM, or of the primary infection that precipitated the EM. Death in the severe forms of EM is often associated with pneumonia. A recent prospective study has shown that treatment of EM major with high-dose steroids at an early stage, with careful monitoring for any evidence of infection and prompt treatment of this, is associated with a better prognosis.

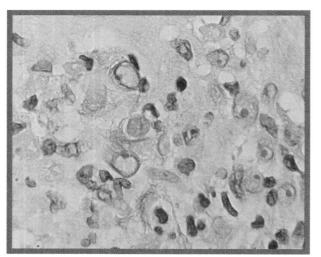

← **Fig. 9.9**
Specific virus induced nuclear changes in keratinocytes allow HSV infections to be diagnosed early. There is a distinctive steel-grey colour centrally, with ring-like accentuation of nucleoplasm at the periphery ('margination of nucleoplasm').

10 | Ulcers and erosions

Case History

The patient, a 49-year-old businessman, had just been made redundant when he developed severe and painful ulceration in his mouth (**Fig. 10.1**). His general practitioner treated him with oral acyclovir and vitamin B, but without success.

Ten weeks later, the patient's symptoms had become so extreme that he was referred as an emergency to the local department of oral surgery. He was finding it increasingly difficult to eat and was rapidly losing weight.

By now the oral ulceration was affecting most of his buccal mucosa, including the tongue and the soft palate. A few recent but extending lesions were also seen elsewhere on the skin (**Fig. 10.2**). The Nikolsky sign was positive.

Biopsies were taken from the patient's oral and skin lesions (**Fig. 10.3**).

→ Fig. 10.1
Painful mouth ulcers, starting suddenly and spreading quickly.

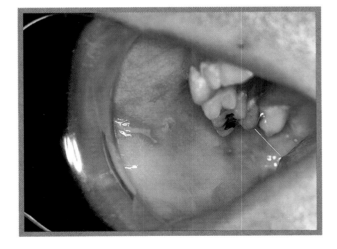

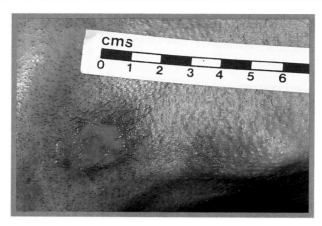

← Fig. 10.2
Painful spreading erosions on the front of the neck.

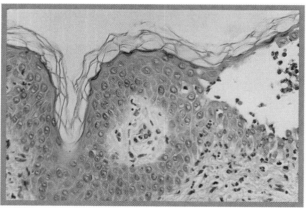

← Fig. 10.3
Skin biopsy of an early lesion, showing that a blister had arisen within the epidermis. Many detached, rounded-off epidermal cells can be seen within the blister cavity.

Questions

1. What is the Nikolsky sign?
2. What is the diagnosis of this patient's condition?
3. Would any further investigations be of value?
4. How should this patient be treated?
5. What is the prognosis?

Answers

1. The Nikolsky sign is positive if sideways pressure on apparently normal skin causes the epidermis to shear off and slide sideways, like wet wallpaper on a wall (**Figs 10.4** and **10.5**). It is characteristic of all types of all types of pemphigus and of toxic epidermal necrolysis. The Russian dermatologist PV Nikolsky described this sign in 1896. It is not the same as a blister extending laterally under pressure – this is less specific and is seen in several other bullous disorders.

2. This patient has pemphigus vulgaris, an uncommon but serious bullous disorder.

    More than half of such cases start with painful oral erosions, which may be present for some months before the onset of a generalised bullous eruption. The initial mouth lesions can easily be confused with other conditions such as erythema multiforme, severe aphthous ulcers, and erosive lichen planus.

    Once the skin lesions appear, the clinical diagnosis becomes easier. The bullae are flaccid and break easily, leaving denuded areas with a collar of detached epidermis at their edges. In the superficial types of pemphigus (erythematosus and foliaceous), blisters may never be apparent clinically (**Fig. 10.6**). Unlike those of pemphigoid (**Fig. 10.7**), they arise on apparently normal skin.

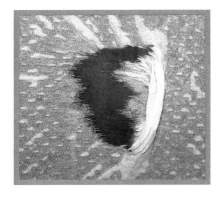

↑ Fig. 10.4
The Nikolsky sign is positive if sideways pressure on the skin causes the epidermis to slide, like wet wallpaper on a wall.

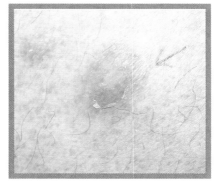

↑ Fig. 10.5
A positive Nikolsky sign in a patient with pemphigus.

3. The histology of pemphigus vulgaris is characteristic – suprabasal blisters with acantholysis (the rounding-off and separation from each other of epidermal cells that have lost their intercellular bridges – see Fig. 10.3). If there are no intact blisters, a smear from an eroded area may be examined for the presence of these acantholytic cells (a Tzanck test).

Pemphigus vulgaris is one of a group of blistering disorders characterised by the presence of IgG autoantibodies directed against the surface of keratinocytes. Their target is a 130 kD polypeptide existing in a molecular complex with plakoglobin, an adhering junction molecule. Direct immunofluorescence of a biopsy specimen increases diagnostic precision and shows IgG deposited between the epidermal cells of both involved and uninvolved skin (**Fig. 10.8**). There is some correlation between circulating autoantibody levels (measured by indirect

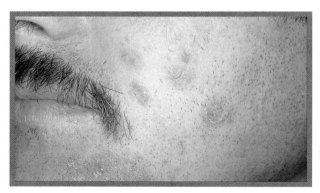

← **Fig. 10.6**
Pemphigus erythematosus: the blisters arise superficially within the epidermis and rupture quickly, leaving crusted erosions.

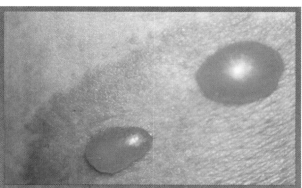

← **Fig. 10.7**
In pemphigoid, the blisters may be tense and often arise on an erythematous base.

immunofluorescence) and disease activity, but treatment should be based on clinical rather than laboratory findings. In pemphigoid, immunoglobulin is deposited along the basement membrane (**Fig. 10.9**).

In most cases, pemphigus vulgaris is not associated with other internal disorders, but a so-called paraneoplastic variant has now been described. Its autoantibodies are directed against an antigen of a higher molecular weight (230kD), and its lesions include an intense and severe stomatitis, which is refractory to treatment, and polymorphic skin lesions that may resemble erythema multiforme. This combination of features should prompt a search for an underlying lymphoma or thymoma.

→ Fig. 10.8
Pemphigus vulgaris: direct immuno-fluorescence shows the deposition of IgG between the epidermal cells, specifically on the hemidesmo-somes.

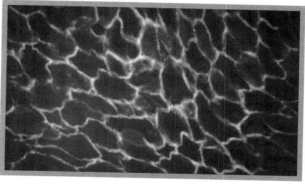

→ Fig. 10.9
In pemphigoid, immunoglobulin is deposited along the epidermal basement membrane.

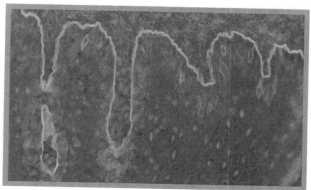

4. The treatment of pemphigus vulgaris is never easy, and has to be tailored to each individual patient.

Most patients are still treated initially with oral corticosteroids, although opinions vary about dosage schedules. As much as 200mg/day of prednisolone may be needed, and, if this fails, plasmapheresis (to remove pathogenetic autoantibodies) or pulsed intravenous methylprednisolone can be used to gain rapid control.

Thereafter, other adjuvant therapies can be introduced, with the aim of cutting corticosteroid intake and side effects, although most carry potentially serious side effects of their own. Of the immunosuppressive drugs, azathioprine and cyclophosphamide are probably the most commonly used. Cyclosporin may be less effective. For highly resistant cases, pulsed intravenous cyclophosphamide can be tried, with or without pulsed intravenous corticosteroids. Long-term immunosuppression leads to loss of fertility and an increased risk of cancer; adjuvant gold therapy may therefore be the first choice in younger patients.

5. Until the early 1950s, patients with pemphigus vulgaris usually died from their disease, with widespread, infected skin lesions and changes in electrolytes and plasma proteins secondary to this. The picture changed dramatically after the introduction of corticosteroids (**Fig. 10.10**): death rates then dropped to a third of their former level – but the use of high doses caused many serious side effects, from which some patients died. Nowadays, the use of adjuvant therapies, mentioned above, with systemic corticosteroids has reduced the 1-year mortality rate to below 10%.

In the present case, the patient at first improved on prednisolone and azathioprine, but within a few months his condition deteriorated. His oral ulcers were particularly hard to clear and remained painful enough to stop him eating a normal diet. Consequently, several other treatments have been tried, in high dosage, both alone and in combination, including systemic prednisolone (at times up to 200mg daily), azathioprine, cyclosporin, intravenous infusions of immunoglobulin, and plasmapheresis. Short-term success has always been followed by relapses.

Side effects have inevitably followed, too: steroid-induced diabetes has been treated with glipiside; osteoporosis with alendronate; a widespread herpes simplex infection with acyclovir; recurrent skin infections with antibiotics; dyspepsia with ranitidine; depression with fluoxetine; and atrial fibrillation with digoxin. Most recently, some success has been achieved with monthly intravenous pulses of cyclophosphamide and methylprednisolone, plus oral maintenance therapy with both. The patient's skin and mouth, however, are still far from clear, and his plasma albumin level remains low.

→ Fig. 10.10
A dramatic fall in mortality from bullous disorders was seen in England and Wales in the early 1950s, when treatment with systemic corticosteroids was introduced.

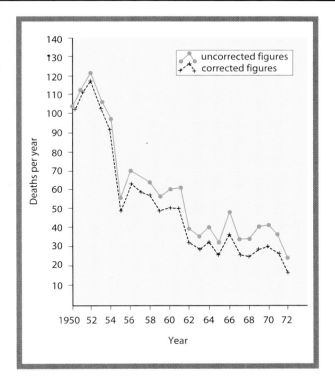

11 | A clue from a condom

Case History

A 68-year-old man had a long history of urological problems. Three years previously, a carcinoma of the kidney had been removed: soon after, he had two further operations for carcinoma of the prostate. Although these operations had been successful, it became necessary for him to have a permanent suprapubic catheter (**Fig. 11.1**), fitted with a special valve, to ensure adequate drainage of his bladder.

These experiences made him worry about the possibility of developing further cancers and he was referred to the skin clinic with a lesion on his nose, thought to be a basal cell carcinoma. It was removed and turned out to be a harmless seborrhoeic keratosis.

At the time of his consultation, he took the opportunity to ask about an itchy rash on his penis (**Fig. 11.2**), present for about 1 year. It had responded, but only partially, to topical steroid applications.

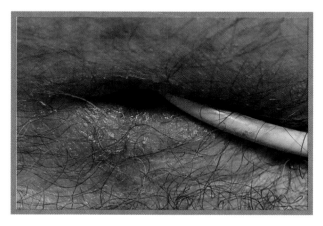

← Fig. 11.1
The skin around the suprapubic catheter quickly became red and itchy.

→ Fig. 11.2
An irritable area also appeared on
the side of the penis.

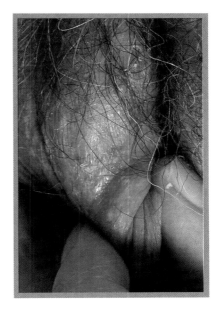

Questions

1. What is the most likely cause of this eruption?
2. Which aspects of his past history should be probed in more detail?
3. Which type of allergy is most likely here?
4. How should this be investigated?
5. What treatment should be given to the patient?

Answers

1. The rash was red, scaly, and itchy: in this area, a chronic fungal infection has to be considered. Scrapings were therefore examined microscopically for the presence of fungal hyphae, which can easily be seen in preparations cleared with potassium hydroxide to which dimethyl sulfoxide has been added (**Fig. 11.3**). This test, however, turned out to be negative.

Other conditions to be considered as causes of a penile eruption include psoriasis (**Fig. 11.4**) and seborrhoeic dermatitis – but the eruption was not typical of these, and there was no trace of them elsewhere. Fixed drug eruptions (**Fig. 11.5**) are not uncommon on the penis, but this patient's lesions did not pass through the typical cycles of activation and remission in relation to taking a particular medication.

The patient had not appreciated that his rash might be related to the indwelling catheter, but an allergic contact dermatitis seemed likely (**Fig. 11.6**).

2. Further questioning was needed on the subject of previous allergies.

Catheters, in general, fall into two classes: homogeneous (made of a single substance such as silicone, PVC, or polyurethane) and heterogeneous (made of a coated substrate). For long-term use, catheters made either of silicone or of coated latex, containing added chemicals, are employed. The latter are the more flexible. The manufacturer of the catheter in question was contacted and said that it was of the coated latex type, and so contact allergy to the rubber component seemed possible.

Contact allergy to rubber itself is rare: most reactions are, in fact, to the various chemicals added to rubber during processing. Soft latex is converted into usable rubber by various vulcanising (curing) agents, which crosslink the polymer chains. Accelerators are chemicals used to speed up this process. Antioxidants are added to stop the rubber perishing in the air. Many of these substances are potent allergens, and the pattern of the rashes they cause is determined by how they are brought into contact with the skin (**Figs 11.7–11.9**).

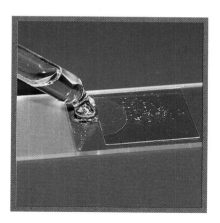

← Fig. 11.3
A solution of potassium hydroxide, to which dimethyl sulfoxide has been added, is run under the coverslip to clear the skin scrapings.

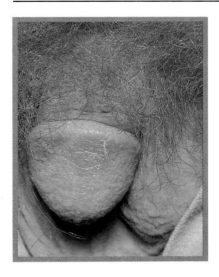

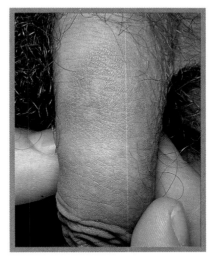

↑ Fig. 11.4
A typical plaque of psoriasis on the penis – sharply marginated and scaly.

↑ Fig. 11.5
The penis is a common site for a fixed drug eruption – here due to tetracycline. This lesion is in the inactive stage of postinflammatory hyperpigmentation.

→ Fig. 11.6
The reactions were confined to the areas where the catheter touched the skin.

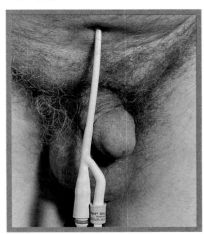

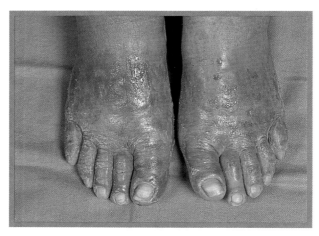

← Fig. 11.7
An allergic contact dermatitis occurring as a reaction to rubber in a pair of slippers.

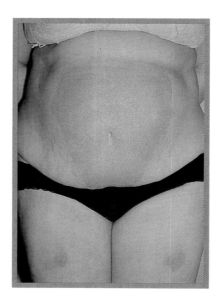

↑ Fig. 11.8
A reaction to an elasticised panel in a corselet.

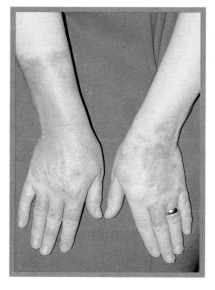

↑ Fig. 11.9
The classic sharp upper margin of allergy to rubber gloves.

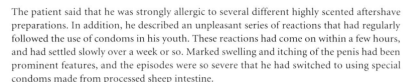

The patient said that he was strongly allergic to several different highly scented aftershave preparations. In addition, he described an unpleasant series of reactions that had regularly followed the use of condoms in his youth. These reactions had come on within a few hours, and had settled slowly over a week or so. Marked swelling and itching of the penis had been prominent features, and the episodes were so severe that he had switched to using special condoms made from processed sheep intestine.

3. The choice lies between 'immediate' and 'delayed' hypersensitivity.

Immediate hypersensitivity is due to reactions to natural rubber proteins, and presents as a contact urticaria (**Fig. 11.10**) that occurs within a few minutes. It is sometimes accompanied by rhinitis, conjunctivitis, and even asthma, especially if powder from rubber gloves becomes airborne.

Delayed hypersensitivity, on the other hand, usually takes a few days to appear, and takes the form of an eczematous type of dermatitis. The appearance of this patient's current penile rash fitted best with this – so, probably, did the history of his reactions to condoms; penile oedema can be a feature of acute contact dermatitis in that area, as well as of contact urticaria.

4. Had the history been more suggestive of contact urticaria, then serum could have been sent for a RAST test to natural rubber latex, remembering that this is not positive in all cases. Prick or scratch tests to extracts from the rubber materials in question require experience and facilities for resuscitation.

In this case, the relevant investigation was skin patch testing to the European Standard Battery of Contact Allergens (**Fig. 11.11**), and the results were read at 48 and 96 hours. This battery includes three main groups of rubber chemical allergens (**Fig. 11.12**). Positive reactions were detected to fragrance mix (as suggested by his aftershave reactions) and to thiuram mix (containing a mixture of three related rubber accelerators). A patch test to a piece of the catheter itself was also positive.

→ Fig. 11.10
Contact urticarial reactions to rubber chemicals, such as shown here, come up immediately; in contrast, contact dermatitis takes a day or two to appear, even in a previously sensitised individual.

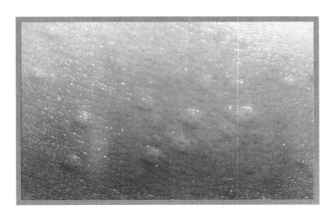

→ Fig. 11.11
The standard battery is supplied at the correct strengths in convenient syringes.

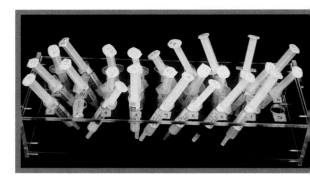

Rubber chemical allergens	
Allergen	**May be found in**
Thiuram mix	Any rubber object: particularly in rubber gloves, elastic, rubber bands, sponges. Also in some fungicides and pesticides. Cross-reacts with disulfiram.
Mercapto mix	Any rubber object: particularly in shoe insoles, some rubber gloves, finger cots, elastic bandages, hot-water bottles, corsetry.
Black rubber mix	Heavy-duty black rubber, e.g. in car tyres, squash balls, rubber handlebars, eyelash curlers. Can cross-react with black hair dye.

↑ Fig. 11.12
Table of the rubber chemical allergens used in the Standard European Patc Test Battery.

These findings fit with the patient's history, as, at one time, thiuram chemicals were the mc common sensitisers in condoms, although this is no longer the case.

5. Delayed hypersensitivity to materials that cause allergic contact dermatitis cannot be reverse by procedures designed to desensitise. Equally, the regular application of topical steroids m partially suppress the condition, but will not cure contact dermatitis while the allergen is st present. In this case, allergen avoidance was achieved by switching to a catheter made solely fro silicone, with no thiuram component. The eruption then cleared quickly and completely.

Striped nails and a furry tongue

12

Case History

The patient had first been seen by a dermatologist at the age of 2 years, with chronic inflammation in his mouth and on his lips. These changes persisted (**Figs 12.1–12.3**), and later his fingernails became crumbly (**Figs 12.4** and **12.5**). Longitudinal brown lines began to appear on his nails (**Figs 12.6** and **12.7**).

→ Fig. 12.1
The patient at the age of 10 years. An adherent, whitish deposit can be seen inside the cheek.

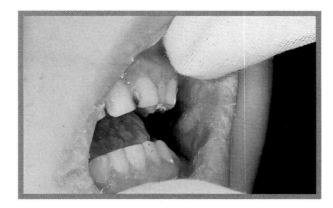

→ Fig. 12.2
Marked angular stomatitis and patchy white depositions on the tongue.

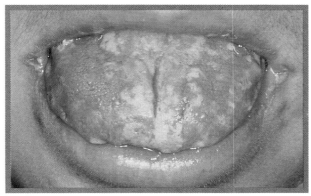

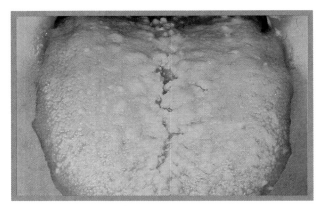

← Fig. 12.3
By the age of 18 years, the white areas on the patient's tongue had thickened and become confluent.

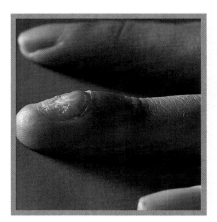

↑ Fig. 12.4
Chronic paronychia has caused persistent swelling of the proximal nail fold. The nail plate itself has become crumbly.

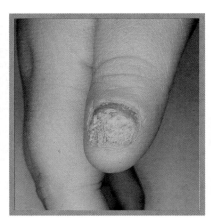

↑ Fig. 12.5
Chronic paronychia and thumbnail dystrophy.

→ Fig. 12.6
Several fingernails began to show striking longitudinal brown lines.

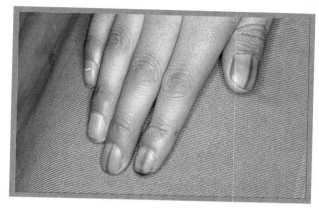

→ Fig. 12.7
Similar brown lines could also be seen on several of the toenails.

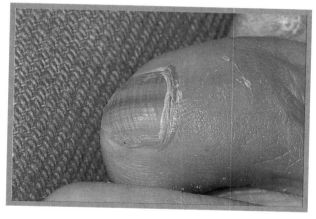

Numerous other health problems have occurred since the first presentation, including repeated chest infections and hypoparathyroidism, requiring the patient to take massive doses of vitamin D from the age of 3 years. Addison's disease was diagnosed after an episode of crisis at the age of 13 (**Fig. 12.8**), and chronic malabsorption has persisted since the age of 14 years. The patient went on to develop insulin-dependent diabetes mellitus at the age of 24 years.

When the patient was 15, he lost hair patchily from his scalp (**Fig. 12.9**), and the bald areas failed to respond to intralesional injections of triamcinolone. More scalp hair was lost, until none was left, and he had to wear a wig.

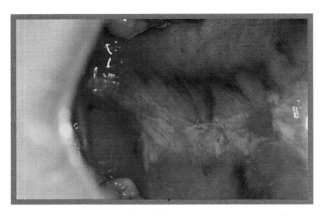

← Fig. 12.8 Pigmentation suggestive of Addison's disease can be seen on the mucous membrane inside the cheek. The whitish deposits remain as before.

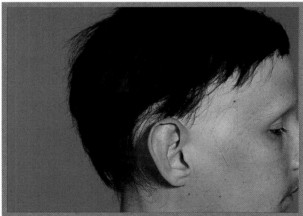

← Fig. 12.9 Patchy hair loss, most marked around the hair margin.

Questions

1. What is the most likely cause of the patient's mouth and nail problems?
2. Is there a single unifying diagnosis here?
3. What are the possible causes of longitudinal pigmented stripes of the fingernails?
4. How would you treat the patient's mouth and nail abnormalities?

Answers

1. This is chronic mucocutaneous candidiasis. Specimens from the adherent white plaques in the mouth grew *Candida albicans*. Microscopy showed hyphae and not just yeast forms (**Fig. 12.10**) – as is usually the case in clinical infection, as opposed to simple yeast carriage. Specimens from the dystrophic nails also regularly grew *C. albicans*, but were negative for dermatophyte fungi.

   C. albicans is an extremely sensitive biological detector of weakness in the body's defense systems. Infections with it range from brief, trivial, surface problems in the otherwise fit, to overwhelming systemic infections. The seriousness of the infection is roughly proportional to the degree to which the host's defenses are compromised. This is seen convincingly in HIV infection. In chronic mucocutaneous candidiasis, the nail folds become red and swollen, and the nail plates thickened and dystrophic. Oral involvement may be accompanied by chronic vulvovaginitis.

   Chronic mucocutaneous candidiasis is a complex diagnostic problem. Sometimes it is associated with other infections, as in severe combined immunodeficiency disease and AIDS. It may also exist as an isolated finding in patients in good general health, with no more than a slight excess of dermatophyte or wart infections, and inconstant underlying defects of cell-mediated immunity. Often there is an associated latent iron deficiency.

   If the condition starts in early childhood, it can be sporadic, or have been inherited either as an autosomal dominant or recessive disorder. Onset in adult life usually signals an underlying disorder such as a thymic tumour, systemic lupus erythematosus, or, most commonly, AIDS. The white ribbed lesions of hairy leukoplakia have sometimes been confused with candidiasis.

→ Fig. 12.10 Scrapings from the mouth lesions, cleared in potassium hydroxide, show candidal pseudohyphae and spores.

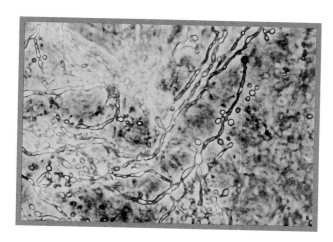

2. This patient has the candidiasis endocrinopathy syndrome (also known as autoimmune polyendocrinopathy–candidiasis–ectodermal dysplasia), inherited as an autosomal recessive trait. Relatives often have minimal changes: this patient's older brother had mild intermittent oral candidiasis only. Oral changes appear first, in early childhood, and the high incidence of organ-specific antibodies, and conditions such as vitiligo and alopecia areata, suggest an autoimmune mechanism for the endocrine abnormalities, too. The combination of hypoparathyroidism and hypoadrenocorticalism is typical of the condition.

3. In a white person, a single dark line running the entire length of one nail (**Fig. 12.11**) is likely to be due to a junctional melanocytic nevus of the nail matrix. Occasionally such lesions change into a malignant melanoma, and at that stage the line may become broader. Multiple pigmented bands affecting many nails are common in non-white persons and are usually of no significance. However, if such stripes appear in a white person, as in this case, Addison's disease should be considered.

4. Systemic treatment is needed permanently both for the mouth and nail lesions, and the candidiasis will inevitably relapse when it is stopped. Both amphotericin B and flucytosine have to be given intravenously, and so are not suitable for long-term maintenance therapy. Oral ketoconazole is effective, although high doses may be needed and idiosyncratic hepatotoxicity is a rare but important complication.

   Itraconazole has several advantages over ketoconazole. It binds only weakly to human cytochrome P450, making it less toxic. It is active against most species of Candida and persists in the tissues – for example, it remains in nail keratin for at least 6 months after the end of treatment. It can be used in doses of up to 200mg daily for at least 3 months in the immunocompromised, and its tissue persistence makes it effective as pulsed therapy – in which one week on treatment is alternated with 3 weeks off. Concomitant administration of astemisole or terfenadine has occasionally led to severe cardiovascular complications and should be avoided. Levels of warfarin, and of phenytoin and oral hypoglycemics, may also be increased by itraconazole.

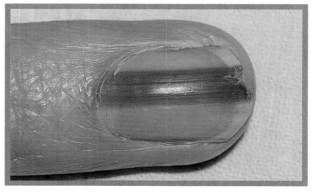

← Fig. 12.11
This broad pigmented line was due to a junctional melanocytic nevus of the nail matrix.

13 | Persistent skin splinters

Case History

A 66-year-old woman had a 3-year history of itchy bumps appearing over her body and limbs (**Fig. 13.1**).

She held strong opinions about their cause, but these varied from time to time. For a while she put the eruption down to a course of nalidixic acid: later she felt that betamethasone cream had helped to keep it going. Her main theory, however, was that the problem was due to an accident during which she had crashed into a wooden door. This, in her view, had embedded large numbers of splinters in her skin. They were still being extruded several years later, and, strangely, even from sites remote from her original injuries.

The lesions remained itchy, and she scratched and picked at them constantly. She was not satisfied with progress and tried to speed things up by spending several hours a day digging out 'splinters' with a sterilised needle. She brought samples of the presumed splinters to the clinic one day (**Fig. 13.2**).These were sent to the laboratory for histological examination (**Fig. 13.3**) – but she was not happy with the subsequent report. A skin biopsy specimen was also obtained (**Fig. 13.4**).

Progress was slow, and she consented to inpatient treatment on two occasions. Each time her skin lesions cleared completely after occlusive bandaging, but swift relapses followed when she left the ward. For a short

→ Fig. 13.1
These itchy, excoriated papules had been present on the trunk and limbs for several years.

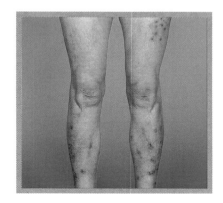

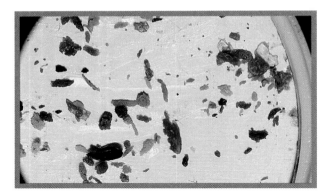

← Fig. 13.2
A selection of specimens brought by the patient to the clinic.

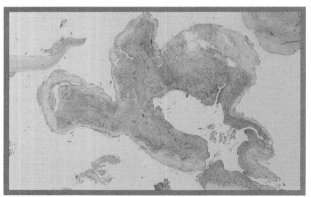

← Fig. 13.3
The 'splinters' were prepared for microscopic examination by the pathology laboratory. This confirmed the presence of epidermis but no splinters.

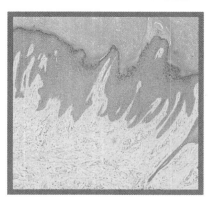

← Fig. 13.4
This slide shows acanthosis (thickening of the epidermis), and psoriasiform hyperplasia.

time she took systemic medication with great success, but the rash soon returned when the patient decided to stop taking the tablets. She no longer attends the skin clinic, preferring to put her faith in homeopathy.

Questions

1. How should the skin lesions be classified, clinically and histologically?

2. How could wooden splinters continue to give so much trouble?

3. What systemic medication was used, and what are its potential side effects?

Answers

1. The lesions are firm, slightly warty, pink nodules, many of which are surmounted by crusted excoriations. They are grouped, and most numerous on the limbs. On morphological grounds, the lesions fit into the category of prurigo nodularis.

The histology fits well with this diagnosis. The epidermis is greatly thickened – with marked hyperkeratosis and acanthosis – and shows striking downward projections. The appearances are those of severe lichenification a term used to describe the thickening of the skin which follows constant rubbing. The histology caused by a wooden splinter is quite different (**Fig. 13.5**). Prurigo nodularis has usually no clear-cut cause. A minority of patients have an associated gluten enteropathy or an underlying pemphigoid. About 80% of patients are atopic. The condition is extremely itchy and tends to persist indefinitely.

→ Fig. 13.5
This microphoto-graph shows a genuine splinter of wood embedded in the epidermis.

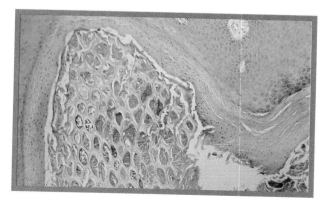

2.   Obviously, splinters cannot behave like this. In this case, the lesions of prurigo nodularis have formed the basis for a series of delusions about the presence of splinters – a variation on the theme of delusions of parasitosis. This is usually a single fixed delusion that is not secondary to any particular psychiatric disorder. Sufferers are often intelligent but rather solitary individuals, sometimes with a medical background. Rarely, the condition is triggered by nutritional deficiencies, cerebrovascular accidents, or schizophrenia. Genuine infestations have always to be excluded (**Figs 13.6** and **13.7**).

Classically, patients bring containers to the clinic with them, thinking that they contain parasites at various stages of development (**Fig. 13.8**). Histology confirms that, as here, only

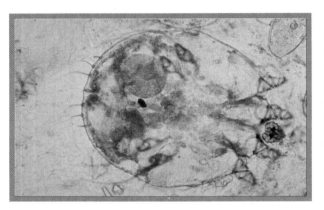

← Fig. 13.6
Scabies has to be excluded. Scrapings from possible burrows should be cleared in potassium hydroxide and examined microscopically. A typical mite and several eggs are seen here.

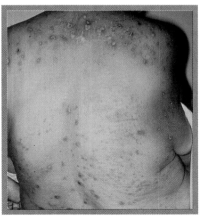

← Fig. 13.7
These lesions, not unlike those of the patient described here, were due to a body louse infestation. Note the sparing of the butterfly area over the scapulae, which the patient could not reach to scratch.

shreds of damaged skin are present. Patients may go to great lengths to purify their skin and its environment: friends and relatives may even be persuaded to join in these activities.

3. Prurigo nodularis and delusional parasitosis are both difficult to treat – their combination makes matters worse. In delusional parasitosis, patients tend to drift from doctor to doctor, complaining about incompetence and looking for physical cures for their disorder. Suggestions that their views on parasites could be mistaken are often greeted with hostility, and followed by failure to reattend.

Direct confrontations are best avoided, as are dogmatic statements that the patient has a mental disorder. Nevertheless, some patients can be persuaded to take medication solely on the grounds that it has helped others with similar problems.

Pimozide was prescribed for this patient. It is probably still the drug of choice, and is usually highly effective. An initial dose of 4mg can be increased slowly, usually to a maximum of 12mg daily. However, it is contraindicated in those with pre-existing prolongation of the QT interval or a history of cardiac arrhythmias. An ECG should be performed before treatment starts, and at regular intervals thereafter in patients on more than 16 mg daily. If repolarisation occurs (prolongation of the QT interval, or T-wave or U-wave changes), the need for continuing the drug should be reviewed. Extrapyramidal symptoms may occur at higher doses.

Compliance is often a problem, and many patients find excuses for stopping treatment once their delusions have settled. Under these circumstances, depot neuroleptics can be used.

→ Fig. 13.8 These 'specimens' do look rather like parasites, but this notion was easily disproved histologically.

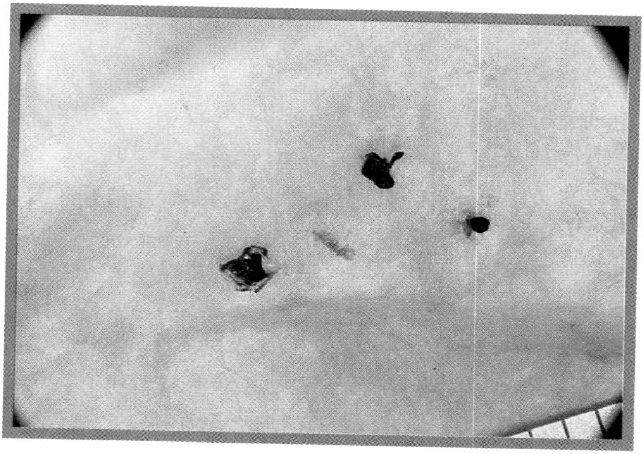

When is a keloid not a keloid?

14

Case History

An abscess arose slowly on the ulnar aspect of the left elbow of a 15-year-old girl, whose past health had included stress-related abdominal pain and mild epilepsy. Her family came originally from Pakistan, but she had not visited that country in the previous 6 years.

The abscess was incised at a local casualty department, and much pus was expressed, although cultures were negative for pathogenic organisms. Nevertheless, apparent clinical sepsis in the area grumbled on, and she was given several antibiotic courses before the abscess finally resolved.

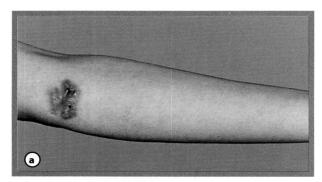
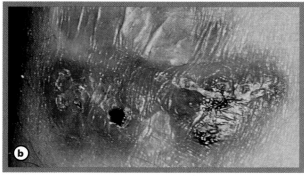

← **Fig. 14.1** Distant **(a)** and close-up **(b)** views of the elbow lesions.

Unfortunately, over the next few months, a painful and ugly raised red–brown area came up at the site of the incision (**Fig. 14.1a** and **b**).

Her family physician took this to be an atypical keloid, and sent her to the skin clinic for an opinion about the best form of treatment. He was surprised to hear later that a biopsy had been taken (**Fig. 14.2**), and that a chest X-ray had been arranged (**Fig. 14.3**).

→ Fig. 14.2
A diffuse lymphohistiocytic infiltrate in the dermis, with granuloma formation.

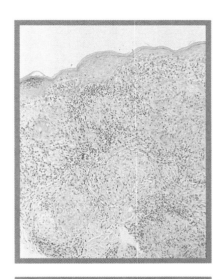

→ Fig. 14.3
A chest radiograph showing several cavitating lesions within the left upper and the right mid-zone, with associated right hilar and paratracheal lymphadenopathy.

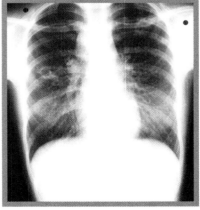

When is a keloid not a keloid?

Questions

1. What is the most likely diagnosis?
2. How could this be confirmed?
3. How should the patient be treated?

Answers

1. Biopsying a keloid is usually a mistake as it can lead to a larger one appearing. However, the borders of this lesion were less well defined than one would expect in a keloid (**Fig. 14.4**) and the haemorrhagic crusting was unusual. In addition, the lesion had arisen to one side of the incision scar, but not on it.

   The dermatologist felt that the lesion was probably a granuloma – a pathological term, but one which also has clinical meaning. A granuloma clinically is a slowly spreading area of chronic inflammation with indurated plaques (**Fig. 14.5**), papules, and even pustules. An important feature is the typical brownish colour, best seen using diascopy (viewing the lesion while it is being pressed on by a glass slide).

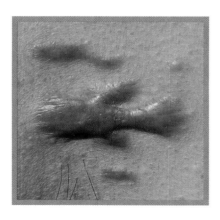

↑ Fig. 14.4
Typical keloids running transversely across the front of the sternum.

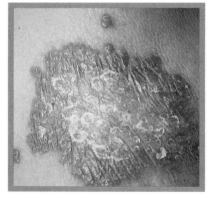

↑ Fig. 14.5
A red-brown well-defined plaque of lupus vulgaris, with scaling and early central clearing.

The biopsy confirmed that there was a florid granulomatous reaction in the dermis, including numerous giant cells, but no evidence of macrophages containing *Leishmania* organisms. This was to be expected, as she had not left the UK during the previous 6 years.

Possible causes of granuloma formation had then to be considered, sarcoidosis, in particular, as it favors scars (**Fig. 14.6**). However, an X-ray of the patient's chest (see Fig. 14.3) showed features suggestive of active tuberculosis.

The elbow plaque, therefore, was an example of lupus vulgaris – a form of cutaneous tuberculosis seen in those who have a moderate or high degree of immunity to the organism.

2. This condition is now rare in the UK, and diagnostic suspicion has fallen as a result. Lesions may be mistaken for psoriasis, Bowen's disease, and even lupus erythematosus. The chief causes of difficulty are leprosy and sarcoidosis, and differentiation may be difficult histologically, too, as the causative mycobacteria may be sparse or not seen at all. Part of the biopsy specimen should be sent for culture for mycobacteria, but a negative culture, as in this case, does not rule out the diagnosis of lupus vulgaris. The tuberculin reaction is usually strongly positive.

3. Untreated lupus vulgaris can progress to cause considerable disfigurement, scarring, and destruction of facial cartilaginous structures. The most serious consequence, however, is the possible development of a squamous cell carcinoma (**Fig. 14.7**).

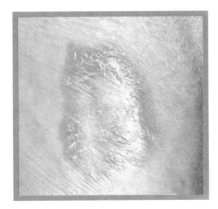

↑ Fig. 14.6
A shiny papery scar present for several years became raised and pink when it was infiltrated by a sarcoid granuloma.

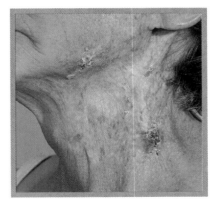

↑ Fig. 14.7
An area of atrophic scarring caused by lupus vulgaris. A squamous cell carcinoma has developed at the lower border of the scar, and an early one on the angle of the jaw .

A full antituberculosis regimen has to be used, even for patients whose tuberculosis is apparently localised to the skin. In this patient, the sensitivity of the organisms isolated from her sputum could be taken into account. She is currently being treated for the first 2 months (the initial phase) with isoniazid, rifampicin, pyrazinamide, and ethambutol. The intention is to continue with only isoniazid and rifampicin for a further 4 months (the continuation phase). Liver and renal function tests were normal before the treatment started and remain so. A good result is to be expected (**Fig. 14.8a** and **b**).

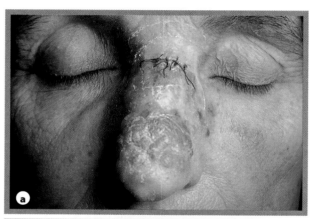

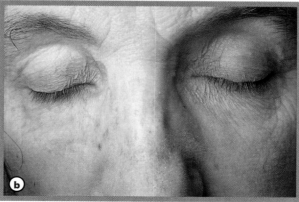

← Fig. 14.8 Another patient, before **(a)** and after **(b)** treatment, whose lupus vulgaris responded fully to a complete course of antituberculous therapy.

Notched nails and a nasty smell

15

Case History

After a spell of hot and sunny weather, a 46-year-old male returned to the dermatology department with an exacerbation of his chronic skin disease. His rash was itchy and beginning to smell unpleasant. His skin problem had started at the age of 16, on the upper back and chest (**Figs 15.1–15.3**), and had spread slowly over the years to involve the scalp (**Fig. 15.4**), ears, arms, and groin. During that time he had developed distinctive changes on the palms and nails (**Figs 15.5** and **15.6**). The patient had been tried on a specific drug, but could not tolerate it, and the drug had to be stopped within 1 month.

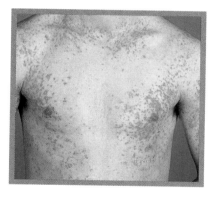

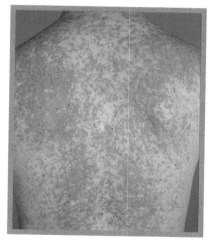

↑ →**Figs 15.1 and 15.2**
Sun triggered this papular eruption on the upper back and chest.

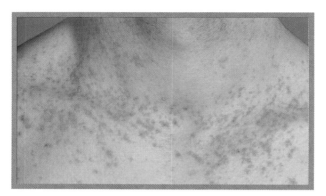

← **Fig. 15.3**
A closer view of the greasy, pink brown papules.

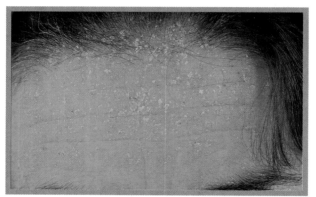

← **Fig. 15.4**
Yellowish scaling on the scalp and forehead.

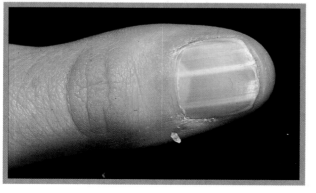

← **Fig. 15.5**
Characteristic nail changes. Red and white longitudinal lines extend from the base of the nail to the free margin, and may terminate in a notch (see Fig. 15.6).

→ Fig. 15.6
A V-shaped notch, present on both nails. Painful longitudinal splits are also common in this condition.

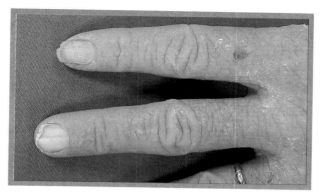

Questions

1. What is the diagnosis ?
2. What complications can occur?
3. Which drug is particularly effective in this condition?
4. What are the side effects of this drug?
5. Which drug exacerbates this condition and psoriasis?

Answers

1. This patient has Darier's disease, a rare disorder of keratinisation that affects both sexes equally and is inherited in an autosomal dominant mode. Skin lesions usually appear between the ages of 6 and 20 years, but rarely as late as 70 years. One-third of patients improve in later life: however, for the majority, the condition is unremitting and chronic.

Itch is common, but malodor is often the most distressing problem. The warty brown papules and plaques appear first on the center of the back and chest, on the scalp, and round the hair margins. Most patients also have scattered papules in their axillae and groins: few have severe flexural disease. Palmar pits and keratotic papules, which interrupt the dermal ridges, occur in most patients, and sometimes are found also on the soles. Small warty papules are often seen on the back of the hand (**Fig. 15.7**). Oral mucosal lesions, most commonly on the hard palate, occur in 15–50% of patients. Heat and sweating provoke outbreaks of the disease, although sunlight aggravates it less consistently.

The histological features of Darier's disease are characteristic (**Figs 15.8** and **15.9**), but the presence of acantholytic dyskeratotic cells in the epidermis is not specific to it. They may also be seen in blistering diseases such as Hailey–Hailey disease/transient acantholytic dermatosis, and in pemphigus. Clefts and lacunae are also seen in the epidermis.

The gene that codes for the mutant protein in Darier's disease lies on chromosome 12q23–24 in all families studied, but the gene differs slightly from family to family.

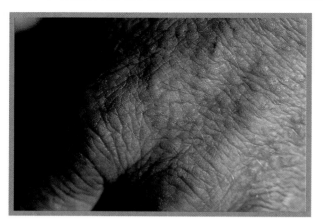

← Fig. 15.7
Innumerable
small warty
papules.

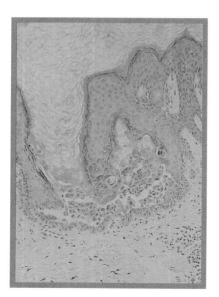

← Fig. 15.8
A focal area of acantholysis can be seen just above the basal layer of the epidermis. Acantholytic keratinocytes can be recognised by their rounded shape and their separation from other keratinocytes. The dyskeratotic nature of these cells is revealed by their brightly staining eosinophilic cytoplasm. Two types of dyskeratotic cells are present: round bodies (see Fig. 15.9) and shrunken bodies (grains: small cells with elongated nuclei and scant cytoplasm) in the cornified layer.

→ Fig. 15.9
Round bodies (corps ronds) are pyknotic nuclei surrounded by dense eosinophilic cytoplasm, between normal epithelial cells.

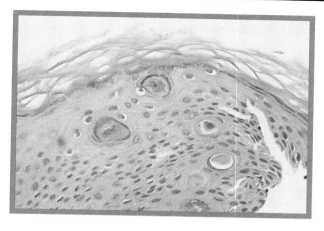

2. Salivary gland swelling is an unusual complication in some families.
   Recurrent localised or widespread cutaneous infections may occur, with *Staphylococcus aureus* and herpes simplex virus being the most common organisms.
   Neuropsychiatric problems such as epilepsy, depression, and mental retardation are more frequent in sufferers from Darier's disease than in the general population.

3. Darier's disease resists treatment with most conventional keratolytic and anti-inflammatory agents. In mild cases, symptomatic relief follows the use of emollients and antiseptics. Topical steroids may help the itch, but have little effect on the course of the disease. The cutaneous manifestations are rather like the follicular hyperkeratosis of vitamin A deficiency, a fact which led to the mistaken idea that the disease was due to vitamin A deficiency. Nevertheless, topical retinoic acid (formed by the oxidation of vitamin A) is sometimes helpful, although its use may be limited by local irritation.

   Oral aromatic vitamin A analogues (retinoids) are of considerable value in treating Darier's disease, but their use is limited by their toxicity. Acetretin, a second-generation retinoid, is now used in place of its predecessor, etretinate. It is contraindicated in women of childbearing potential unless effective contraceptive measures are used. Acetretin is less lipophilic, and has a half-life of 50–60 hours, as compared with the 120 days of etretinate. However, etretinate has been identified in plasma samples from some patients treated with acetretin, so a contraceptive period of 2 years is still needed after therapy is completed.

   Retinoids bind to multifunctional nuclear receptors (retinoic acid receptors) which are members of the steroid/thyroid superfamily. Once the ligand binds, receptor molecules influence the regulatory sequences of cellular DNA and modulate gene expression. Retinoids have complex effects and the mechanism of their action in hyperproliferative disorders is not precisely understood. However, they generally modulate cell proliferation and inhibit epidermal cell growth and differentiation.

4. The adverse effects of acetretin are dose related, although the alopecia depends also on the duration of therapy. Mucocutaneous reactions are common: drying of the mucous membranes of the eyes, nose, and lips, and cheilitis occur in most patients. Other symptoms include alopecia, desquamation, and pruritus. Changes in lipid profile are often observed, and hypertriglyceridemia is particularly common. Liver enzyme levels may also become raised and there are potential long-term effects on bones. Spurring and ossification of ligaments mimic diffuse idiopathic skeletal hyperostosis (**Fig. 15.10**).

   Although 90% of patients improve with retinoids, only 50% continue with them long-term, as many prefer the disease to the side effects of the drugs, coupled with the inconvenience of hospital attendances and blood tests. Doses of 30–50mg/day are effective.

5. Lithium exacerbates Darier's disease, possibly by increasing cell proliferation, and has even been known to trigger it. Its effect on psoriasis is better known. As with Darier's disease, lithium can exacerbate and trigger psoriasis, and make it resistant to treatment. Lithium reduces brain inositol levels by inhibiting inositol monophosphatase. In addition, inositol levels in some peripheral tissues fall after lithium treatment. Inositol does not cross the blood brain barrier, therefore supplementation with inositol antagonizes some of the peripheral side effects, but not its central beneficial effects. Concomitant treatment with inositol, essentially a food supplement, may be a worthwhile as a nontoxic adjunct to the treatment of patients with psoriasis on lithium.

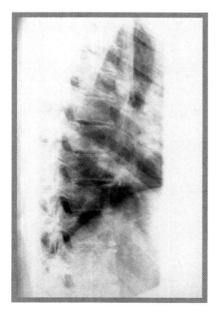

← Fig. 15.10
Bridging osteophytes and syndesmophytes are present at multiple levels.

Rapidly progressive
16 | nasal ulceration

Case History

An 84-year-old woman on a psychogeriatric ward with senile dementia was referred to the dermatology department with a small ulcer on the left nasal ala. This was initially thought to be a cigarette burn aggravated by picking. A skin biopsy showed coagulative necrosis of the epidermis, suggestive of injury with an exogenous agent, but no evidence of a neoplastic or granulomatous process (**Fig. 16.1**). Within a month she had been sent to the Ear, Nose and Throat department from Accident and Emergency, with recurrent episodes of bleeding from the ulcer (**Fig. 16.2**). A further biopsy showed the same features seen in the first biopsy.

She then failed to keep several follow-up appointments over the following 3 months, but her ulcer continued to enlarge. Tissue loss then accelerated alarmingly (**Fig. 16.3**), and she was referred by the ENT surgeons to an oncology department for consideration of chemotherapy, with a provisional clinical diagnosis of Stewart's lethal midline granuloma. Only then was it realized that she had undergone transection of the trigeminal nerve 30 years previously for trigeminal neuralgia.

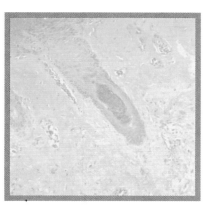

← Fig. 16.1
This skin biopsy shows coagulative necrosis of the epidermis, with no evidence of an underlying malignant or inflammatory process.

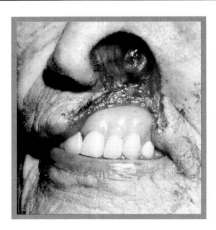

↑ Fig. 16. 2
At this stage, ulceration of the wing of the nose was advancing rapidly.

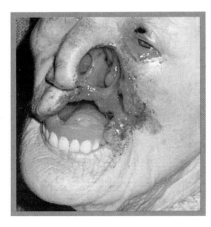

↑ Fig. 16.3
The tissue loss has now become gross – note progression to involve the orbit.

Questions

1. What was the real cause of this nasal ulcer?
2. What conditions had to be ruled out by a skin biopsy?
3. How would you manage this patient?
4. What else might give rise to this syndrome?

Answers

1. This patient has the trigeminal trophic syndrome, which most commonly follows transection of the peripheral sensory fibers of the trigeminal nerve, or injection of phenol into the Gasserian ganglion. These treatments were used once to treat trigeminal neuralgia, now more commonly managed with transcutaneous electrical stimulation (TENS). Patients often develop paresthesiae, with burning, creeping, or crawling sensations focusing attention on the area, and picking follows, as an attempt to relieve these unpleasant sensations. Characteristically, an initial small crust develops into a crescentic ulcer on the nasal ala (**Fig. 16.4**), and may gradually extend to involve the cheek and upper lip. The tip of the nose is typically spared, possibly because of the an overlap in innervation from the first and second divisions of the trigeminal nerve, and there is usually inflammation in the surrounding tissue.

2. It was important to rule out the following:

(a) Malignancies:

Basal cell carcinoma (BCC). This is the most common skin tumour in Caucasians and arises on the head and neck in the majority of cases. Early lesions are commonly pearly or translucent, with telangiectasia and a rolled edge (**Fig. 16.5**). Ulceration is usually a late event, but BCCs that ulcerate early, particularly those involving the nasolabial fold, behave aggressively.

Squamous cell carcinoma (Fig. 16.6). This is another common skin tumour in Caucasians, which may arise *de novo* or from premalignant conditions such as actinic keratoses or Bowen's disease. It often develops on sun damaged skin, and induration is the earliest clinical sign. It may be ulcerated, plaque-like, or verrucous, and the borders are usually ill defined.

(b) Granulomatous conditions such as:

Wegener's granulomatosis (WG). A clinicopathological triad of necrotizing granulomatous vasculitis of the upper (**Fig. 16.7**) and lower respiratory tract, and glomerulonephritis. Skin involvement occurs in 40–50% of patients, as purpura, nodules, haemorrhagic bullae, and pyoderma gangrenosum-like lesions. Localized WG, confined to the nose, has been described, and the antineutrophil cytoplasmic antibody (ANCA) test is both sensitive and specific for the condition.

Gumma – a syphilitic swelling with a tendency to ulcerate. This usually starts in the subcutis and extends through the dermis into the epidermis. Lesions vary in size from 2–10cm, and have a punched-out appearance, favoring sites such as scalp, face, chest, palate, and legs. Gumma differs from congenital syphilis – the latter produces a saddle-shaped appearance to the nose and is commonly associated with characteristic tooth changes (**Fig. 16.8**).

→ Fig. 16.4
Another example of the trigeminal trophic syndrome, at a relatively early stage.

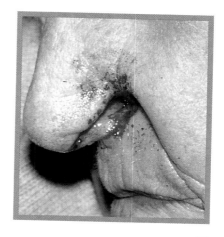

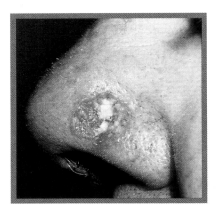

↑ Fig. 16.5
An ulcerating basal cell carcinoma on the nasal ala. BCCs have a predilection for the nose.

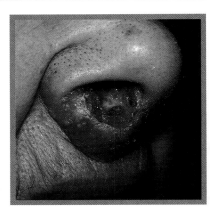

↑ Fig. 16.6
This bulky ulcerated tumour of the nostril was a squamous cell carcinoma.

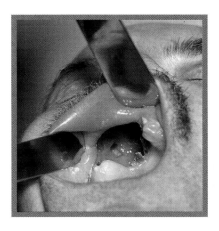

↑ Fig. 16.7
An example of Wegener's granulomatosis – an ulcerated area can be seen within the nostril.

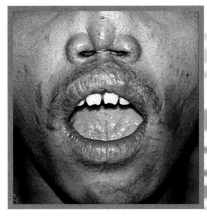

↑ Fig. 16.8
The saddle-shaped nose and notched incisors of congenital syphilis.

Lupus pernio – this relatively common cutaneous manifestation of sarcoidosis typically presents as large bluish red or violaceous nodules or plaques on the nose, cheeks, ears, or hands. Nasal involvement is more or less symmetric (**Fig. 16.9**) and is associated with swelling, ulceration, or crusting of the nasal vestibule.

South American leishmaniasis (espundia) – immunity develops too late in this form of leishmaniasis to prevent blood-borne metastasis of the parasites to the mucosa of the nose, mouth, palate, and larynx. The nasal septum, rather than the alae, is a site of predilection.

Rhinoscleroma – this chronic, slowly progressive, potentially fatal, infectious and mildly contagious disease is caused by the bacterium *Klebsiella rhinoscleromatis*. At first localized to the nasal fossae, it then invades the upper respiratory tract, where it produces an infiltrating granuloma with a marked tendency to sclerosis and subsequent obstruction (**Fig. 16.10**).

(c) The lymphoproliferative disorders: Stewart's lethal midline granuloma (now thought to be a T-cell lymphoma) and lymphomatoid granulomatosis. These are related to angiocentric, angiodestructive lymphoproliferative processes, now included under the term 'angiocentric immunoproliferative lymphoma' (AIL), and are regarded as lymphomatous. Clinically, the predilection of AIL for midline nasopharangeal structures rather than the nasal alae should distinguish it from the trigeminal trophic syndrome. Histologically, AIL shows a mixed cellular infiltrate, with small lymphocytes and variable numbers of large, atypical lymphoid cells, of T-cell lineage. This contrasts with the nonspecific and rather sparse inflammatory change seen in ulcers associated with the trigeminal trophic syndrome.

3. The management of patients with the trigeminal trophic syndrome, particularly if they are older or demented, is notoriously difficult. Infection can be minimized by topical antibacterial agents, with intermittent courses of systemic antibiotics for episodes of cellulitis. Further trauma can be limited by simple dressings, the use of a face mask, or elbow extension splints or gloves. Centrally acting agents such as carbamazepine or benzodiazepines should be

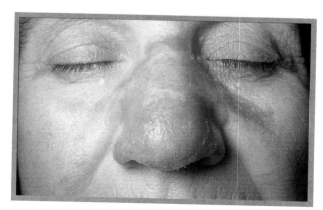

→ Fig. 16.9
The swollen nose of lupus pernio — here red–brown, but usually more plum coloured. External ulcerations seldom occur.

considered if the patient is anxious or agitated; and iron supplements if recurrent bleeding is a problem. Prostheses fitted by plastic or dental surgeons have been tried with some success, and, more recently, rotation of a flap from the innervated unaffected side of the midline to cover the defect has been described. There has been one report of successful treatment with TENS.

4. Conditions that affect the trigeminal nucleus in the pons or spinal tract, such as the posterior inferior cerebellar artery syndrome or syringomyelia, are less common causes of this syndrome. Light touch and pain, in addition to temperature, should be tested in the area served by the three divisions of the fifth cranial nerve (**Fig. 16.11**). Sensory deficits may occasionally involve the periphery of the face while sparing the central area, and vice versa.

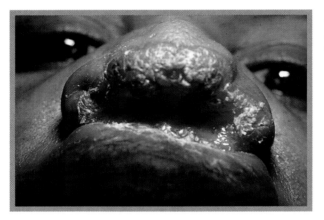

← Fig. 16.10
A severe example of rhinoscleroma.

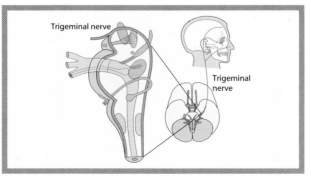

← Fig. 16.11
The spinal tract of the fifth cranial nerve extends from the pons to the lower medulla.

17 | Sunny side up

Case History

An 84-year-old man had a 2-year history of a progressive itchy redness on his face and forearms, worsening after sun exposure. A diuretic, prescribed for hypertension, appeared to have aggravated but not caused the rash. In the past, he had had dermatitis on his hands for several years, and thought he was allergic to chrysanthemums (**Fig. 17.1**). During his thirties, he had spent several years in the tropics with the Royal Air Force.

On examination, the patient had a florid rash over the face (**Fig. 17.2**), neck, forearms, and hands (**Fig. 17.3**), with a sharp cut-off. A number of investigations were performed (**Fig. 17.4**), including a skin biopsy. In addition, some specific tests were arranged to establish the diagnosis.

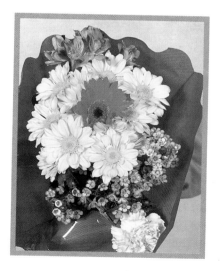

↑ Fig. 17.1
The patient thought that he developed an eruption on his hands whenever he came into contact with chrysanthemums, his favourite flowers.

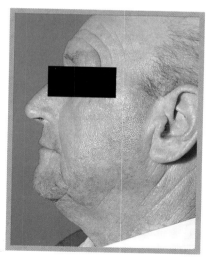

↑ Fig. 17.2
A chronic, thickened, and intolerably itchy eruption of the face.

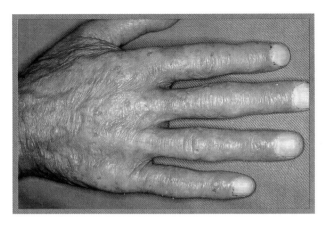

← Fig. 17.3
The backs of the patient's hands were also affected.

Investigations	
FBC:	Normal, apart from an eosinophil count of 0.4%
ANF:	Negative

← Fig. 17.4
Table of investigations.

Questions

1. What is the most likely diagnosis?
2. Could the diuretic have exacerbated the problem?
3. How would you confirm your clinical diagnosis?
4. How would you manage this condition?

Answers

1. **Fig. 17.5** lists some of the conditions to be considered in a photosensitive patient.
    The diagnosis here is chronic actinic dermatitis (also known as actinic reticuloid, 'reticuloid' implying a histological similarity to a reticulosis). The main histological feature is a dense lymphocytic perivascular infiltrate in the upper and mid dermis. Dermal oedema and extravasated red blood cells are also seen. This is a severe, chronic, and persistent form of photosensitivity, which usually affects middle-aged and elderly males. Affected and unaffected skin of these patients is extremely sensitive to both UVB (280–314nm) and to UVA (315–400 nm), and sometimes to visible light. Consequently, they react to light that has passed through glass or clouds. These reactions occur at lower than normal radiation doses (**Fig. 17.6**). Patients often fail to realize that they are photosensitive, as the lesions develop hours or even days after exposure to light, and the photosensitivity is so severe that the rash never clears totally. The diagnosis is based on a high index of suspicion, and phototesting. These patients often have multiple contact allergies, including fragrances and oleoresins derived from plants.

	Causes of photosensitivity
Condition	**Features**
Polymorphic light eruption	Common, itchy rash appears within hours or days of sun exposure (see Fig. 17.6). Worst in spring and improves with tanning.
Drug-induced photosensitivity	Causes include amiodarone, nalidixic acid, phenothiazines, tetracyclines, and thiazides.
Chronic actinic dermatitis	Affects elderly men who react to light even when it has passed through window glass. Also often allergic to plant oleoresins.
Phytophotodermatitis	Due to the psoralen content of certain plants, e.g. giant hogweed.
Porphyrias	Most commonly porphyria cutanea tarda in heavy drinkers. Blisters, hypertrichosis, and skin fragility in exposed areas.
Other skin conditions	Those aggravated by light include lupus erythematosus, herpes simplex, Darier's disease, and xeroderma pigmentosum.

↑ Fig. 17.5
Table showing some causes of photosensitivity.

2. Yes, the diuretic could have exacerbated the problem. Diuretics such as hydrochlorothiazide (**Fig. 17.7**) and frusemide are well-known causes of phototoxic reactions. Other drugs can cause them, too (**Fig. 17.8**). Photosensitivity may persist for many months after withdrawing the drug. Furthermore, it may not always be possible to discontinue treatment with photosensitizing drugs.

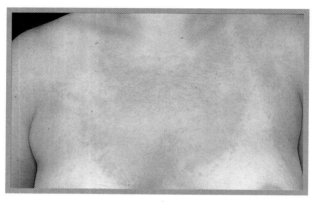

← Fig. 17.6
A view of a polymorphic light eruption. The confluent and papular erythema spares the sites protected from the sun under the patient's swimsuit and under her chin.

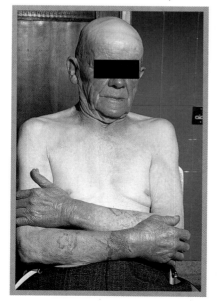

← Fig. 17.7
A thiazide diuretic induced this reaction. The patient's cap protected his scalp, and his shirt his trunk.

with amiodarone, for example, there may be no satisfactory alternative. A broad-spectrum sunscreen containing titanium dioxide or zinc oxide must then be used, as virtually all drug-induced photosensitive rashes are produced by wavelengths within the UVA range. Photoallergic reactions are sometimes produced by topically applied agents, such as suncreens themselves, which often contain the photosensitizer para-aminobenzoic acid (PABA) and PABA esters, or by perfumes containing musk ambrette.

Most plants are harmless when in contact with the skin, but a few, particularly compositae and members of the lichen family, can cause irritant, allergic or phototoxic reactions (**Fig. 17.9**).

→ Fig. 17.8
This florid, vesicular, sharply defined phototoxic eruption was attributable to griseofulvin.

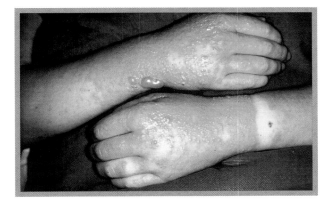

→ Fig. 17.9
The area of skin against which the plant had rubbed became inflamed after exposure to sunlight. This streaky appearance is typical of a phototoxic reaction.

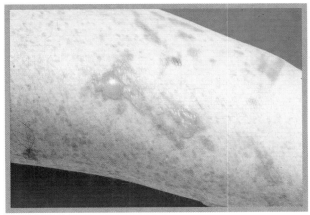

3. Patients with a suspected photosensitive rash such as actinic dermatitis should ideally be investigated with irradiation skin tests using broad-spectrum, particularly solar-simulating, sources, which may induce the eruption. Narrow waveband or monochromatic irradiation studies can be used to define the action spectrum of some conditions.

Chronic actinic dermatitis is defined photobiologically by the experimental provocation of spongiotic dermatitis with UVB, and frequently by longer wavelengths, in the absence of a photoallergen ('spongiosis' means intercellular oedema in the epidermis). These patients are so photosensitive that eczematous lesions can be induced in virtually all cases by phototesting. Patch testing (**Fig. 17.10**) and phototesting (**Fig. 17.11**) are also indicated in eczematous photosensitivity, and may identify an inducing or exacerbating allergen. Sunscreens, in particular, are increasingly recognized as a cause of contact dermatitis; this is clearly relevant in photosensitive patients. The allergen may be the sun filter, the perfume, or the preservative. These tests should be performed only after the measures discussed below have controlled the dermatitis.

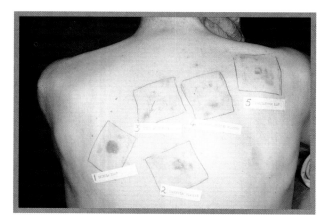

← Fig. 17.10
This patient is showing a 2+ and 3+ reaction to crysanthumums and primula plants.

4. If the rash is severe, admission to hospital is wise. The patient should be nursed in a room with Uvethon-Y screens on the windows, so that all UV light is screened out. Topical steroids and sedating oral antihistamines will also alleviate the symptoms. Once discharged, patients should apply the topical steroid first, followed by a sunscreen 10 minutes later, first thing in the morning and again in the early afternoon. Tinted sunscreens containing titanium dioxide are now available. If the rash occurs despite using such sunscreens, Uvethon-Y screens should be placed on the windows of the rooms the patients use most at home. Patients should remain indoors, even with sunscreen on, between 10 a.m. and 3 p.m., as UVA is at its strongest then. Tightly woven protective clothing should also be worn. Occupational exposure to UV should also be considered (arc welding and fluorescent tubes if not protected with a plastic diffuser). If patients fail to improve, immunosuppressive agents such as azathioprine or cyclosporin may be indicated.

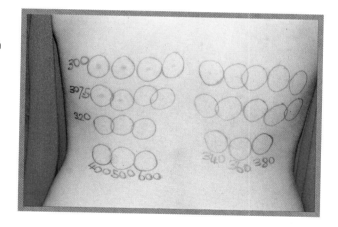

→ Fig. 17.11 This patient has been tested with a mono-chromator light source. This is used to determine the specific wavelength of ultraviolet radiation to which a patient is sensitive.

A surgical cure of
18 itching

Case History

A 60-year-old female, a retired teacher, was referred to the skin clinic with a persistent generalized itch, present for about a year. At first a new washing powder had been blamed, but reverting to the old one had made no difference. The patient's general practitioner had treated her with trimeprazine for itching, and twice for scabies, but with no success.

Her general health was good; she was a nonsmoker who drank no alcohol. Her past history included reactions on her hands to scented soap.

On examination, there was no evidence of scabies, or indeed of any specific skin disease, although scratch marks were visible over her trunk, sparing the area over her scapulae (**Fig. 18.1**), and on her lower legs. Her liver was palpable and she had palmar erythema (**Fig. 18.2**), but no sign of leukonychia or the 'half-and-half' nails of chronic renal failure (**Fig. 18.3**). However, her nails were highly polished (**Fig. 18.4**). She was not clinically jaundiced. The results of a variety of tests are shown in **Fig. 18.5**.

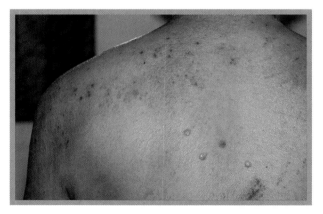

← Fig. 18.1
Notice the way the scratch marks avoid the areas of skin over the scapulae.

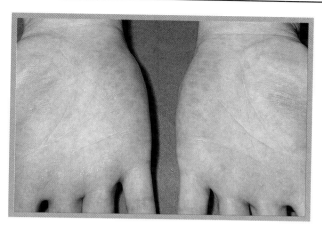

← **Fig. 18.2**
The patient showed bilateral palmar erythema.

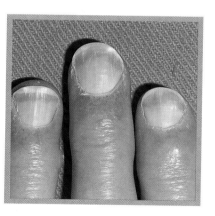

↑ **Fig. 18.3**
The proximal part of the nail is pale and the distal part is pink: the telangiectasia of the proximal nail fold is due to systemic lupus erythematosus.

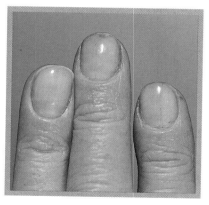

↑ **Fig. 18.4**
Remorseless rubbing and scratching has buffed the nails to a high polish.

Test results	
Test	**Results**
FBC:	Hb 14.2g/dl, ESR 46mm/h., WBC 6.3 × 10⁹/l
ANF:	Negative
Bilirubin:	38mmol/l
ALT:	104u/l
Alkaline phosphatase:	501u/l
γGT:	270u/l
Blood urea:	3.9mmol/l
Thyroxin:	131mmol/l
Viral hepatitis screen:	Negative
Autoantibody tests to smooth-muscle and mitochondria:	Negative
Chest X-ray:	Normal

← Fig. 18.5
Table of results of relevant tests in this patient.

Questions

1. Which important causes of itching should be considered here?
2. How would you investigate this patient?
3. How do you interpret the results of these investigations?

Answers

1. Pruritus is a symptom with many causes. The first step must always be to check thoroughly for the presence of a surface cause. In this patient there was no obvious sign of a skin disorder, but well-known traps include scabies, and dermatitis herpetiformis – in which the diagnostic small, grouped blisters are quickly broken by scratching. Itching after a bath can be due to detergents in bubble baths, to polycythemia, or to aquagenic pruritus. Over washing and dryness of the skin contribute to the common 'winter-itch' of the elderly: the physical signs are often trivial, even when there is marked itching. A positive butterfly sign (see Fig. 18.1) suggests an internal cause for itching and is due to an absence of rash or scratch marks on an area of the back that cannot be reached (**Fig. 18.6**).

The physical examination of this patient raised the possibility of liver disease in which itching signals biliary obstruction. Itching is infrequent in infective hepatitis, but may be an early warning of primary biliary cirrhosis. Other causes include intrahepatic cholestasis caused by some drugs (e.g. chlorpromazine and testosterone). Although not relevant in this case, itching in pregnancy may sometimes be due to cholestasis, although the detectable abnormalities of liver function are often minimal.

Some important internal causes of itching, which should be considered in every case, are listed in **Fig. 18.7**. Itching is a feature of chronic, but not of acute, renal failure. It is rare in carcinomatosis, but common in Hodgkin's disease, often occurring long before any other manifestations of the disease. Despite the assertions in many textbooks, generalized pruritus is a rare presentation of diabetes.

→ Fig. 18.6
Elderly people cannot reach the skin in the scapula area and so cannot scratch it.

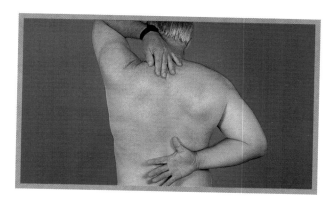

→ Fig. 18.7
Table of some internal conditions that can cause generalized pruritus.

Conditions
Liver disease
Renal failure
Internal malignancy
Polycythemia
Iron deficiency
Neurologic disease
Thyrotoxicosis
(Diabetes)

2. A full general examination is needed before any tests are performed. Look particularly for the puncture marks of drug addicts, the stigmata of liver disease, the enlarged lymph nodes, liver, and spleen of the reticuloses, and for thyrotoxicosis, and anemia.

If there are still no clues, from either the history or the clinical examination, and the itching is severe, consider using a reasonable battery of screening tests, such as those listed in **Fig. 18.8**.

The results of the relevant tests in this patient are shown in Fig. 18.5. In view of these, the patient was referred to the Liver Unit for further investigations, including an abdominal ultrasound, a CT scan of the abdomen (**Fig. 18.9**), and a percutaneous transhepatic cholangiogram (**Fig. 18.10**).

3. The most important abnormalities were in the liver functions tests – confirming the findings of the physical examination. The greatly raised alkaline phosphatase level suggested biliary obstruction, but provided no evidence as to the site of that obstruction. The raised γGT level also fitted with biliary obstruction, as did the raised ALT level, although also introducing the possibility of damage to liver cells. At that stage, the most likely diagnosis on clinical grounds was thought to be primary biliary cirrhosis, but the absence of autoantibodies to smooth muscle, and in particular to mitochondria, made this unlikely.

Abdominal ultrasound is an important initial investigation in biliary obstruction: here, the hepatic parenchymal echo pattern was normal, but there was both intrahepatic and extrahepatic dilatation of the biliary tree. The gallbladder was large, but no calculi were seen

Investigations
Chest X-ray
Urine for protein and glucose
Liver function tests
Blood urea and creatinine
Serum iron
Hemoglobin, ESR, and WCC
Serum thyroxin
Plasma proteins and electrophoresis

↑ Fig. 18.8
Table of tests suitable for the investigation of unexplained pruritus.

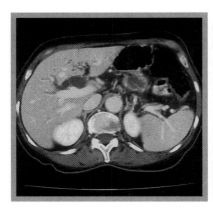

↑ Fig. 18.9
CT scan showing dilation of the intrahepatic, pancreatic and common bile duct.

in it. The pancreas was somewhat bulky. A CT scan showed dilatation of the intrahepatic, pancreatic, and common bile ducts (see Fig. 18.9). In percutaneous transhepatic cholangiography (see Fig. 18.10), contrast material is injected, under radiological control, through a fine-bore needle into an intrahepatic duct. This confirmed biliary obstruction and revealed that the obstruction was at the level of the ampulla of Vater. A malignant obstruction was one possibility. An endoscopic retrograde cholangiopancreatography was therefore attempted. A firm swelling was found at the ampulla, but seemed to be covered by normal duodenal mucosa. Indeed, biopsies showed a normal duodenal villous structure, with no evidence of neoplasia, but brushings from the ampulla itself showed clumps of atypical cells thought to be suspicious of malignancy (**Fig. 18.11**).

At laparotomy, an annular pancreas was found, surrounding the second part of the duodenum. The ampulla of Vater was a little prominent, but no tumour could be felt. Wedge biopsies were taken and sent for frozen section examination. The changes found were those of a small, moderately differentiated adenocarcinoma, and it was decided to perform a radical pancreatoduodenectomy, as suspicious lymph nodes had been found near the greater curvature of the stomach. Histology of these glands showed no evidence of tumour, however. The patient recovered well from the operation, and is still well 5 years later.

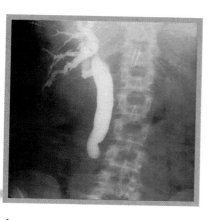

↑ Fig. 18.10
Percutaneous transhepatic cholangiography confirmed biliary obstruction at the level of the ampulla of Vater.

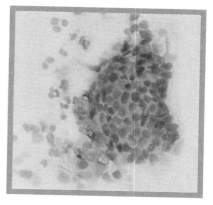

↑ Fig, 18.11
The cytological features of the brushings from the ampulla of Vater confirm malignancy with pleomorphism and hyperchromatic staining of the nuclei.

An ulcer to be kept
19 | away from the surgeons

Case History

A 45-year-old woman presented with a 1-week history of a rapidly extending ulcer on the left knee. This had started as a large painful 'blood blister', ulcerating within 24 hours, and visibly enlarging each day over the next week (**Fig. 19.1**). She had had deforming rheumatoid arthritis (**Fig. 19.2**) for many years, for which she had received a variety of systemic agents including myocrisine, hydoxychloroquine, and methotrexate. A number of investigations were performed (**Figs 19.3** and **19.4**).

The diagnosis was established and appropriate systemic treatment was commenced. Marked improvement was noted within 3 days.

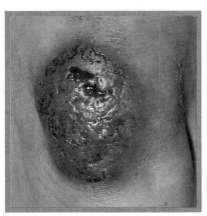

← Fig. 19.1
Serosanguinous material exudes through a number of small openings (cribiform) in this massive inflammatory swelling.

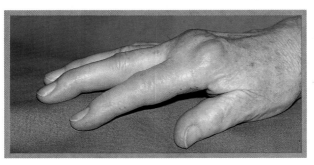

← Fig. 19.2
Deforming rheumatoid arthritis.

→ Fig. 19.3
Table of
investigations.

Investigations	
FBC:	Neutrophil leukocytosis $(14.7 \times 10^9/l)$; otherwise normal
ESR:	69mm/h
Serum protein electrophoresis:	Faint IgG-λ monoclonal band
Biochemical screen:	Normal
Rheumatoid factor:	Positive
Autoantibody screen:	Negative
Chest X-ray and skeletal survey:	Normal
X-ray of hands:	Erosive arthropathy (see Fig. 19.4)

→ Fig. 19.4
There is
generalised loss
of bone density
in a periarticular
pattern aound
the meta-
carpophalangeal
(MCP) joints.
Bone erosions
are well seen in
the left index
MCP joint.

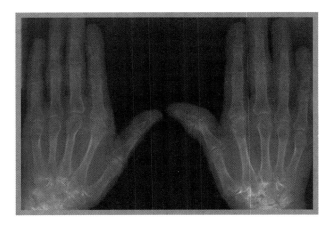

Questions

1. What is the diagnosis?
2. Is a skin biopsy diagnostic?
3. How would you treat the condition?
4. What are the implications of the monoclonal gammopathy?

Answers

1. This patient has pyoderma gangrenosum (PG). This is characterized by rapidly progressive ulcers with a characteristic appearance. Classic lesions start as a pustule on a red base (**Fig. 19.5**), or as a red nodule or plaque that rapidly enlarges and ulcerates. Features that distinguish PG clinically from other ulcers include the liquefying center without eschar formation; the purple, inflamed, undermined border (**Fig. 19.6**); and a more peripheral red border with a necrotic, haemorrhagic base. The other ulcer that progresses at this rate is seen in patients with necrotizing fasciitis (**Fig. 19.7**) and they are much more severely ill. Deep fungal infections or vasculitis should be considered when the progress is slow. In addition, diseases such as a cutaneous lymphoma may rarely mimic PG.

    Patients with PG are often admitted to a surgical unit. Unless the disease is recognized, wide surgical debridement may be undertaken, which only causes a further progression of the disease at its margins. Pathergy is well recognized in PG: lesions then develop at sites of trauma including intramuscular injections.

    About half of patients with PG have associated chronic inflammatory disease such as rheumatoid and rheumatoid-like arthritis, inflammatory bowel disease [Crohn's disease (**Fig. 19.8**) or ulcerative colitis], malignancies of the haemopoetic system, paraproteinemias, and chronic active hepatitis. Treating the systemic disease often, but not always, improves the PG lesions.

    An atypical, superficial, bullous form of PG is recognized (**Fig. 19.9**): all of the original cases died within 6 months of presentation with a rapidly progressive leukaemia. The form of PG in these patients differed from typical PG histologically, by the superficial nature of the process and by the lack of necrosis and liquefaction, and clinically, by their more subdued skin colour

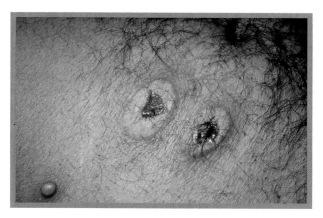

← Fig. 19.5
The early pustular stage of pyoderma gangrenosum.

(blue–grey) and the extending bullous reaction. Many cases of bullous PG have now been documented, usually in association with a hematological malignancy arising *de novo*, or when polycythemia rubra vera transforms into acute leukaemia. This variant of PG is therefore an ominous sign. Bullous PG lesions may be single or multiple, and show no sex or age predilection. A rapid response to prednisolone therapy is usual, and scarring is rare because of the superficial nature of the process.

→ Fig. 19.6
The undermined purple border is distinctive.

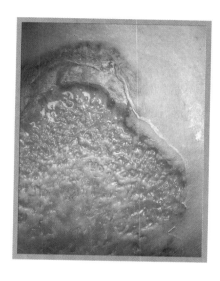

→ Fig. 19.7
Necrotising fasciitis: within 24 hours a small but tender area of perineal inflammation spread to this extent. The patient survived, but only after emergency surgery.

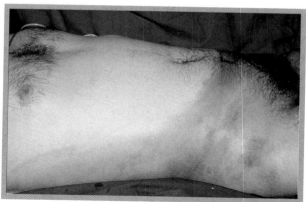

Atypical forms of PG and Sweet's syndrome (SS) have developed simultaneously in a patient with myeloid metaplasia. PG and SS share a number of characteristics, including the presence of an intense dermal neutophil infiltrate, pathergy, and the rapid responsiveness to immunosuppressive therapy. The term 'neutrophilic dermatosis of myeloproliferative disorders' has been proposed, to combine these two entities into a single diagnosis. Some think this should even be broadened to 'acute neutrophilic dermatosis', to include cases with no hematological disturbance.

2. Histopathological features of PG are characteristic but not diagnostic. A predominantly neutrophilic superficial and deep perivascular and interstitial infiltrate is typically seen in the dermis. Neutrophils often fill the infundibulum of a hair follicle, leading to the suggestion that PG begins as a suppurative folliculitis. Vasculitis is rare in PG and when it occurs, appears to be secondary to the primary process.

The pathogenesis of both PG and SS is unknown. Their association with diseases in which circulating immune complexes are present might suggest a pathogenesis similar to the mechanism proposed for necrotizing vasculitis. However, although direct immunofluorescence shows immunoreactants (e.g. IgM, IgG, and C3) in dermal blood vessels in PG and SS, there is little evidence of circulating immune complexes or complement abnormalities. Alteration of neutrophil function has been reported in both conditions, but with some contradictory results, making it difficult to draw definite conclusions.

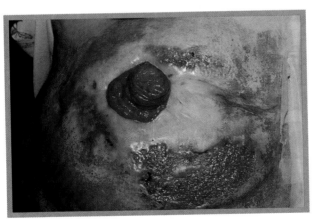

← **Fig. 19.8**
Extensive pyoderma gangrenosum in a patient with severe Crohn's disease and an ileostomy.

3. The most important part of management is to recognize the disease early, before much destruction has taken place. Systemic steroids are the mainstay of therapy and should be started in high doses. Most patients will respond to 60–80mg of prednisolone daily – it is better to suppress the process quickly than to start too low and end up with ever higher doses. When the dose is sufficient, the lesions will become quiesent within 24 hours. After 3–4 days, the daily dose of prednisolone can often be reduced, at first quite rapidly (by 20mg every 3–4 days), and then more slowly, depending on response. Some patients require low doses on alternate days for months or even years. Dapsone, a drug known to inhibit neutrophil cytotoxicity, is often useful as a steroid sparing agent. Other drugs reported to be effective include intralesional steroids, cyclosporin, and minocycline.

4. The association of PG with monoclonal gammopathy, mostly of the IgA isotype, is well documented. It is unclear whether this association has any prognostic significance, and it may simply reflect an altered immune status, as a number of associated immune abnormalities have been described in PG. Malignant progression of the monoclonal gammopathy is unlikely, but biannual serum protein electrophoresis may be prudent.

→ Fig. 19.9
A superficial, bullous form of pyoderma gangrenosum.

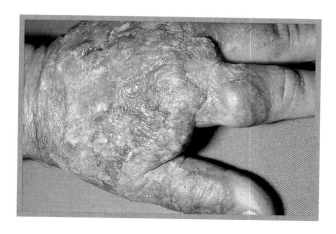

Pink patches and
20 | purple nodules

Case History

A 29-year-old male developed flat pink lesions on the front of his chest; they became raised and purple over the next few months (**Fig. 20.1**). There was no history of trauma and he was on no medication other than a weak topical corticosteroid for persistent seborrhoeic dermatitis on his face and trunk. He had lost weight over the previous year and had experienced two episodes of pneumonia.

A skin biopsy was taken, and special staining was performed.

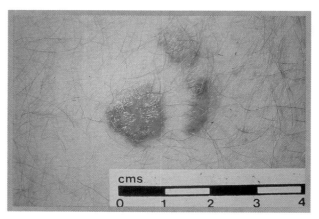

← Fig. 20.1 Although there is some pigmentation, the purple background is distinctive.

Questions

1. What is the diagnosis? What special stain was used?
2. How would you treat this condition?
3. What are the other skin manifestations of the underlying disorder?

Answers

1. This patient has Kaposi's sarcoma (KS). There is still debate over whether this is a malignancy of endothelial cell origin or a hyperplastic response to human herpesvirus 8. Kaposi's sarcoma begins as subtle pink macules, which darken with time as haemosiderin is deposited. Some lesions arise at sites of trauma (Köebnerization), and can simulate an insect bite, a dermatofibroma, a pyogenic granuloma, or, in the later stages, lichen planus or a melanoma. Four clinical forms of KS are recognized:

    (i) The classic form – this affects elderly males of eastern European or Mediterranean origin, and usually involves the lower legs, progressing slowly proximally (**Fig. 20.2**).

    (ii) A more rapidly progressive African variety – here, lymph node involvement is predominant and skin lesions are unusual (**Fig. 20.3**).

    (iii) Post-renal transplantation – KS may develop following renal transplantation (about 3% of patients), but resolves after immunosuppressive therapy has been stopped.

    (iv) The AIDS-associated form – this is seen predominantly among homosexual HIV-positive patients, although the proportion of patients presenting with KS and AIDS is now decreasing. Distal oedema can precede visible lesions. At presentation, half of the patients have oral lesions usually fixed, red, submucosal plaques on the hard palate or gums. Progression of the KS is determined by the immune status of the patient.

    Silver stains should be performed to rule out bacillary angiomatosis (discussed later).

→ Fig. 20.2
This elderly male developed an increasing number of purple nodules over many years, with associated lower-leg oedema.

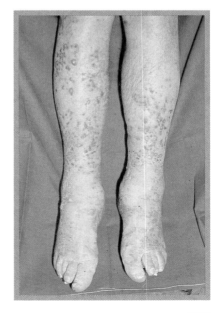

2. Individual lesions can be excised or treated with cryotherapy. Radiotherapy is the treatment of choice for painful or swollen lesions, or nodular disease of the extremities. Disseminated disease can be treated with interferon, interleukin-2, or chemotherapy. Zidovudine can also help – suggested mechanisms of action include improved immunity, a cytotoxic effect on KS cells, and suppression of human herpesvirus 8.

3. The skin is involved at some stage of HIV infection in at least 85% of patients, and the signs of progression towards AIDS are often cutaneous and include a host of opportunistic infections and other inflammatory disorders (**Fig. 20.4**). Some of these – for example, herpes

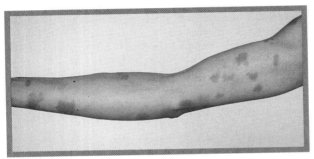

← Fig. 20.3
Within weeks of arriving in the UK, having emigrated from East Africa, this patient developed numerous purple brown patches on the trunk and limbs.

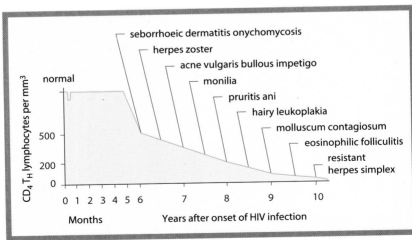

↑ Fig. 20.4
Skin manifestations of HIV disease depend on the degree of immunosuppression, as determined by the CD4 count.

simplex and zoster infections, folliculitis, and seborrhoeic dermatitis – often occur in healthy individuals; whereas others – for example, KS, oral hairy leukoplakia (**Fig. 20.5**), and bacillary angiomatosis – are almost pathognomonic of HIV infection. An excess of drug reactions is related to high prevalence of the slow acetylator phenotype. The Stevens–Johnson syndrome and toxic epidermal necrolysis are also seen more frequently in HIV-positive patients.

Regarding infectious diseases (viral, bacterial, fungal, or infestations), a high level of clinical suspicion is necessary if these are to be diagnosed early enough for management to be effective. Atypical manifestations are common, and rare organisms are often found. Early biopsy, with the use of special stains and tissue culture, is advisable, preferably before starting treatment.

The first manifestation of an HIV infection is the seroconversion reaction. It is characterized by headache, fever, pharyngitis, profound malaise, lymphadenopathy, and a fine morbilliform rash on the trunk, chest, back, and upper arms. The rash may resemble pityriasis rosea (although this more typically takes up a 'T-shirt' distribution), syphilis (which has a more profound systemic upset, patchy hair loss, and a polymorphic rash with papules and plaques), glandular fever, erythema multiforme (often accompanied by suffusion of the face and an identifiable triggering factor in some 50% of cases), and, lastly, a drug eruption (which may have a more widespread distribution). The seroconversion reaction lasts 4–5 days, with recovery apparently complete within 1 week. Patients are highly infectious during this time and the CD4 cell count may plummet to 200 cells/ml and then rebound. Zidovudine has been used with variable results.

Herpes simplex virus (HSV) infections can be confusing in HIV disease, because patients are also susceptible to other ulcerating disorders. Chronic HSV infection (**Fig. 20.6**) may lead to tumour-like, crusted ulcers or a verrucous, persistent ulceration on a digit. A Tzanck smear, culture, or biopsy will confirm the diagnosis. Oral and genital HSV infections usually respond to acyclovir, but, if they do not, a switch to foscarnet sodium (Foscavir) should be considered.

→ Fig. 20.5
Oral hairy leukoplakia is pathognomonic of HIV infection. Unlike in candidiasis, these vertical white streaks cannot be shifted with a spatula.

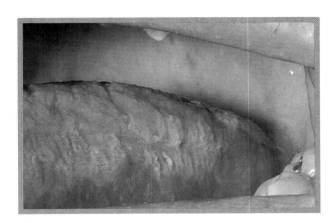

Varicella-zoster virus (VSV) infection is often an early manifestation (**Fig. 20.7**). Verrucous, hyperkeratotic, and crusted plaques can persist for weeks. Postherpetic neuralgia, unusual in healthy patients under 65 years of age, can follow. Treatment should be with high-dose acyclovir (800mg 4-hourly) until the crusts have been shed (10–12 days). HIV-positive patients with a past history of chickenpox may develop sparse atypical lesions, suggesting a reactivation of endogenous virus: those previously unexposed to VZV have a severe primary illness with malaise and pneumonitis.

Molluscum contagiosum is one of the most common viral infections associated with HIV disease, usually in those with CD4 counts of less than 200 cells/ml. Lesions can be large (**Fig. 20.8**), up to 1 cm in diameter, and are often on the face and mantle area. They may simulate cryptococcosis or histoplasmosis, but these are symptomatic and tend to occur in patients with CD4 counts of less than 50 cells/ml. Biopsy will differentiate between them.

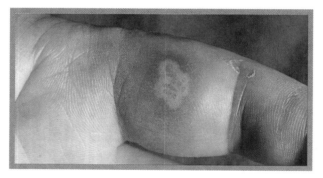

← Fig. 20.6
This persistent herpes simplex infection on the finger has not reached the chronic verrucous stage.

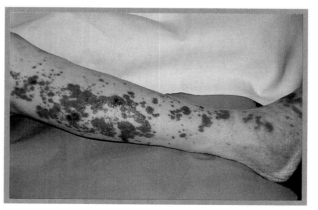

← Fig. 20.7
Be suspicious of HIV infection if the zoster covers three or more adjacent dermatomes, skips to disparate dermatomes, or is accompanied by severe toxicity.

Genital and anal warts (caused by human papillomavirus) are common in patients with AIDS, and HIV infection renders all warts more prolific and difficult to treat. Perianal condylomata can reach an alarming size – such lesions should arouse suspicions of HIV seropositivity.

Bacterial infections are common in HIV disease. Diminishing cell-mediated immunity and macrophage function lead to a loss of protection against species of *Salmonella*, *Listeria*, and *Mycobacteria*. Later, B-cell and neutrophil dysfunction allows organisms to invade through the skin and mucosae, especially if breached by intravascular catheters.

Staphylococcus aureus is the most common pathogen in HIV disease, causing folliculitis, impetigo, ecthyma, and secondary infection of breached skin.

In bacillary angiomatosis (BA), pyogenic granuloma-like vascular nodules proliferate in the skin and subcutaneous tissues. They are due to organisms of the genus *Bartonella* (formerly *Rochalimea*). *Bartonella henselae* is responsible, in healthy individuals, for cat-scratch disease, and *B. quintana* causes bacillary angiomatosis. The organisms can be seen, with the Warthin–Starry silver stain, as tangled masses or as single organisms lying between the proliferating blood vessels. Affected patients have moderate to advanced HIV disease, and the multiplicity of lesions is due to bacteremic seeding. Lesions can be solitary or widespread, on the face, trunk, or extremities. They are red, purple, or flesh coloured, and range from a few millimeters to several centimeters in diameter. KS may resemble BA, but KS lesions are more often multiple and are often found on the head. Patches, plaques, and nodules (**Fig. 20.9**) are the primary lesions of KS, in contrast to BA, in which cystic, pedunculated, eroded, and crusted lesions are often seen. Treatment with erythromycin or doxycycline, for at least 4 weeks, is usually effective.

Many AIDS patients (about 30%) have a history of syphilis (caused by *Treponema pallidum*), and syphilitic ulcers can facilitate the transmission of HIV. Serology may be falsely positive or negative, and so dark field microscopy is the diagnostic test of choice. Syphilis can follow an accelerated course, with the tertiary stage being reached within months. Patients are no longer infectious 48 hours after starting antibiotic therapy.

→ Fig. 20.8
Mollusca are typifed by their umbilication.

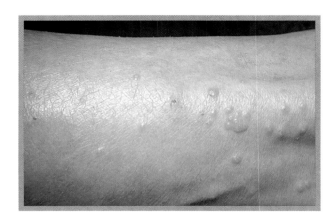

The cutaneous lesions of systemic mycobacterial infections may be nondescript and even indistinguishable from folliculitis. A skin biopsy will confirm the diagnosis. Skin lesions are seldom the only clinical manifestation. In advanced HIV disease (CD4 count <50cells/ml)), *Mycobacterium avium-intracellulare* (MAI) may be the most common cause of disseminated bacterial infection, but it still is rare.

With dermatophytes, unusual presentations must be expected: for example a grossly hyperkeratotic type of tinea pedis simulating psoriasis. Both *Trichophyton rubrum* and *Epidermophyton floccosum*, the most common organisms, respond to terbinafine treatment. Tinea versicolor and pityrosporum folliculitis are especially common in HIV-infected individuals (**Fig. 20.10a** and **b**), and the high prevalence of seborrhoeic dermatitis supports the view that *Pityrosporum ovale* is a major etiological factor in these conditions. Seborrhoeic dermatitis is seen in about 10% of the normal population, but in 70% of HIV-positive patients, even in the early stages (**Fig. 20.11**). It may respond to topical corticosteroid and antifungal agents, but some patients require systemic ketoconazole or fluconazole, sometimes indefinitely.

Mucocutaneous candidiasis, without an obvious cause, should raise the possibility of an HIV infection. Relapses after treatment reflect increasing immunodeficiency.

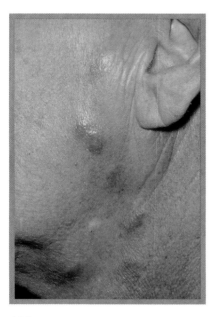

← Fig. 20.9
This patient sought treatment for his multiple, nodular Kaposi's lesions because they were easily seen and socially stigmatising.

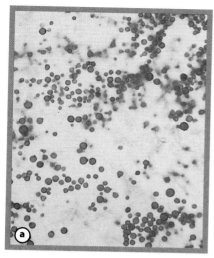
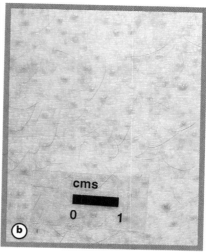

↑ Fig. 20.10
Pityrosporum yeasts make up a part of the normal skin flora **(a)**, but increased colonisation in hair follicles of the immunosuppressed patient causes a folliculitis **(b)**.

→ Fig. 20.11
Seborrhoeic dermatitis, often extensive, is a frequent early manifestation of HIV infection.

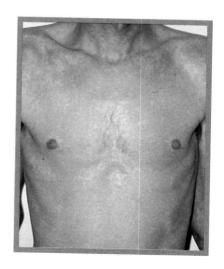

An example of cryptococcosis is shown in **Fig. 20.12**. Although this yeast, *Cryptococcus neoformans,* has a predilection for the brain and meninges, the skin is occasionally involved, and the prevalence of infection with this agent in AIDS patients in the UK is 4%. Primary skin infections occur, but the respiratory tract is the usual portal of entry for this fungus, which normally exists as a saprophyte. Cutaneous and mucous membrane lesions occur in about 10% and 3% of cases, respectively. The most common cutaneous lesions are usually firm or cystic, slow growing, subcutaneous erythema nodosum-like swellings.

HIV patients can carry an unusually heavy load of scabies mites, while experiencing little pruritus. Mites are easily seen in skin scrapings, and treatment with 5% permethrin is effective, though recurrences are common.

Eosinophilic folliculitis, a noninfective disorder, affects the face, neck, upper trunk, arms, and back. Tense pustules with erythematous halos develop, but are rarely seen intact as they are so itchy. Scabies should be ruled out. Histology shows an inflammatory infiltrate with eosinophils clustered within and around hair follicles. The cause is unknown, but many patients respond to UVB phototherapy or to oral itraconazole or metronidazole.

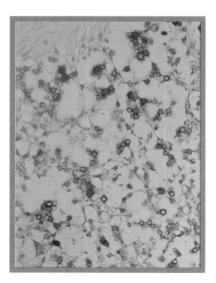

← Fig. 20.12
These encapsulated budding cells in a mesh of connective tissue typically produce a minimal inflammatory reaction.

The prevalence of Reiter's syndrome, another noninfective disorder, is increased in patients with AIDS. However, it is still not clear whether this is due to immune dysregulation, to primary or secondary viral effects, or to an increased exposure to triggering infective agents. Keratoderma blenorrhagicum usually appears 1–2 months after the onset of arthritis and conjunctivitis. The soles are always involved, and the backs of the hands, feet, digits, and nails are commonly affected too. Reiter's syndrome can mimic psoriasis (**Fig. 20.13**), which is treatment resistant in HIV disease.

The prognosis for patients with AIDS has improved dramatically over the past 12–18 months. Many now use triple therapy (generally consisting of two nucleoside analogs and a protease inhibitor), as drug-resistant strains emerge in the face of incomplete suppression of replication. The goal of treatment should be maximal suppression of replication for as long as possible. Treatment is recommended essentially for all persons with CD4 cell counts <500×10⁶/l, or with CD4 cell counts >500×10⁶/l and active viral replication (>10000 viral copies/ml). However, some experts advise treatment for HIV-positive patients with CD4 cell counts >500×10⁶/l and any detectable level of virus.

→ Fig. 20.13 Reiter's disease but you would be forgiven for thinking this patient had psoriasis.

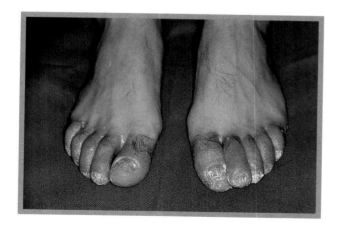

21 | Shades of King George

Case History

At the age of 30 years, this male patient had sought medical advice for recurrent and painful blisters on sun-exposed sites **(Fig. 21.1)**. The blisters healed slowly to leave scars, and his skin seemed to be abnormally fragile. A number of investigations, including a skin biopsy **(Fig. 21.2)** and urinalysis, were performed.

The diagnosis was established, and over the next 5 years the patient managed to avoid alcohol and underwent a regular procedure that was effective in controlling his condition. However, he then started drinking

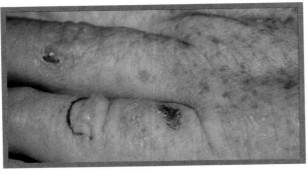

← **Fig. 21.1**
At age 30: the blister on the little finger is to be biopsied, and the numerous milia are due to subepidermal blistering.

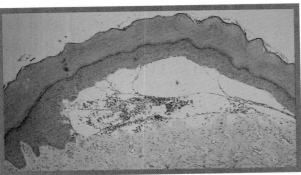

← **Fig. 21.2**
A skin biopsy showing a subepidermal blister, above a dermis that is almost devoid of an inflammatory cell infiltrate, with solar elastosis.

again, and was lost to follow-up until he presented 25 years later (**Fig. 21.3**) with a history of weight loss over the previous 3 months and intermittent abdominal pain. Further investigations, including a CT scan (**Fig. 21.4**), revealed a solid intra-abdominal lesion. Resection of this mass (**Fig. 21.5**) was uncomplicated, but he died of pneumonia 4 months later.

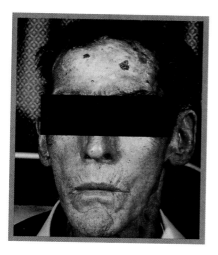

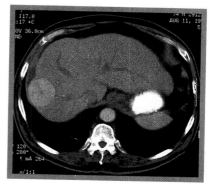

↑ Fig. 21.3
Heavily sun-damaged pigmented skin with crusting and erosions most marked on the forehead.

↑ Fig. 21.4
This CT scan (in the arterial phase) shows a hypervascular mass with a central scar in the liver. There is a small amount of ascites and the liver has an irregular surface, consistent with cirrhosis. The diffuse enhancement of the hypervascular mass would suggest a hepatoma. A hemangioma would typically show peripheral enhancement.

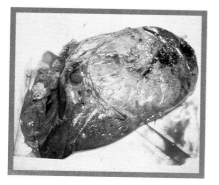

← Fig. 21.5
The gross appearance of the resected hepatic mass.

Questions

1. What was the original diagnosis?
2. What are the main features of this condition and how would you investigate it?
3. What would you expect to find in the liver and skin biopsies?
4. Has any infective agent been linked to this condition?
5. Was the abdominal mass related to the original diagnosis?
6. How would you manage the blistering?

Answers

1. The original diagnosis was porphyria cutanea tarda (PCT). This is the most common type of porphyria, which comprises a heterogeneous group of disorders; either acquired (sporadic or type I), or inherited (familial or type II) as an autosomal dominant trait. Both types share a reduction in hepatic uroporphyrinogen (URO) decarboxylase activity. Some 80% of cases are sporadic, and the remaining 20% are familial. Most people who inherit the enzyme defect do not develop PCT.

Sporadic PCT requires additional factors (**Fig. 21.6**) to become symptomatic.

Most male patients with sporadic PCT drink excessive amounts of alcohol, and up to a third of these develop cirrhosis. Alcohol and estrogens may also precipitate the familial type of PCT. Iron plays an important role in the pathogenesis, too: an hepatic iron overload is present in nearly every case of PCT, and plasma iron is raised in up to 50% of patients.

Factors
Fasting
Liver disease (usually alcohol induced)
Liver transplantation
Estrogens
Iron
Polyhalogenated cyclic hydrocarbons

← Fig. 21.6
Additional factors required for porphyria cutanea tarda to become symptomatic.

2. Familial PCT can present at any age, including childhood, whereas the the sporadic type usually starts in the third decade of life or later. Typical cutaneous signs include vesicles and bullae, appearing on sun-exposed sites and taking many weeks to heal. The resultant scars often show milia (see Fig. 21.1) and may be atrophic. Increased pigmentation, or sometimes mottled hypopigmentation, may be seen, and scleroderma-like white or yellow plaques appear, most commonly on the chest. Patients often notice an increase in skin fragility, and facial hypertrichosis, which develops insidiously and is more prominent in women (**Fig. 21.7**). Porphyrin levels are increased in the plasma, urine, liver, and feces. Typically, levels of uroporphyrin I and III are increased in the urine and plasma. Fecal levels of isocoproporphyrin –and, sometimes, coproporphyrin, 7-carboxylate porphyrin, and urophyrin – are typically raised also. The iron concentration in the plasma and in the liver is increased.

Pruritus is often troublesome. In monochromator studies, light of the same wavelength as that absorbed by the porphyrin molecule (400 nm) (**Fig. 21.8**) has been shown to cause skin lesions in the porphyric patient. Hepatomegaly is common in PCT, and liver function tests are abnormal in nearly all cases. There is a 25% prevalence of diabetes mellitus, and there appears to be an association with systemic lupus erythematous and chronic active hepatitis. Urine can be examined for a coral-pink fluorescence under a Wood's light (**Fig. 21.9**). The sensitivity of the test can be increased by acidifying the urine, or by adding talc, which absorbs porphyrins and allows the fluorescence to be seen more clearly.

→ Fig. 21.7
This female patient with porphyria cutanea tarda has hypertrichosis on her cheeks.

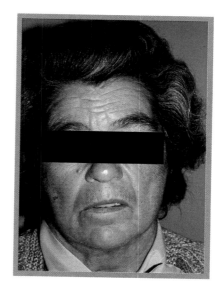

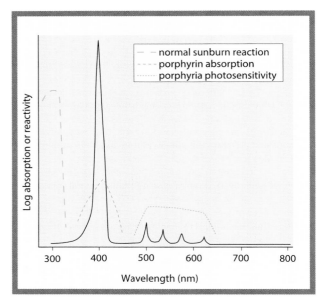

← Fig. 21.8
The action spectrum for light absorption of the porphyrias.

- — normal sunburn reaction
- ‑ ‑ porphyrin absorption
- ··· porphyria photosensitivity

Log absorption or reactivity

300   400   500   600   700   800
Wavelength (nm)

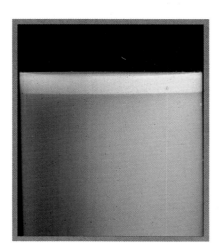

← Fig. 21.9
The typical coral-pink fluorescence of urine under a Wood's light. This may be negative if the skin lesions are resolving at the time.

A few patients on chronic haemodialysis develop PCT, but 'pseudoporphyria' is more common in this group – although their lesions resemble PCT clinically, their porphyrin levels are normal. Another form of pseudoporphyria, with PCT-like blistering and skin fragility, is seen in fair-skinned individuals with a history of excessive sun exposure and the use of sunbeds. Drugs such as tetracyclines, nalidixic acid, frusemide, naproxen, and sulfonamides can also provoke the condition.

3. The skin biopsy shows a subepidermal bulla and a minimal inflammatory infiltrate in the dermis. Venules and capillaries in the upper dermis are frequently rimmed with a homogeneous, eosinophilic, PAS-positive material. This rim is also seen in erythropoietic porphyria, and tends to be wider in that condition. Immunostaining with anti-type-IV collagen demonstrates 'caterpillar bodies' in the roof of the blister. When PCT arises on nonexposed sites, where there is solar elastosis, it can be difficult to differentiate histologically from other subepidermal blistering diseases such as acquired epidermolysis bullosa. In PCT, the liver always contains increased amounts of porphyrin. Liver biopsy shows haemosiderosis in at least 80% of cases, variable fatty change, inflammatory infiltrate, necrosis, and granuloma formation.

4. Recent studies have detected a high prevalence of hepatitis C (HCV) markers in patients with the sporadic, but not the familial type of PCT. The prevalence of HCV infection in these patients varies from 95% in southern Europe, to 10% in Ireland, and 18% in the Netherlands – all higher than in the general population in these areas. The presence of asymptomatic abnormalities supports the view that HCV-related liver disease is the cause of sporadic PCT. Certainly, HCV-related liver disease, and some other liver diseases, can trigger symptomatic PCT in the genetically predisposed. Whatever the mechanism, HCV infection should always be looked for in patients with sporadic PCT.

5. Patients with PCT have an increased risk of developing hepatocellular carcinoma. Hepatic tumours are usually associated with chronic hepatitis or liver cirrhosis, but there is some evidence that the development of PCT may also occur as a paraneoplastic phenomenon secondary to hepatocellular carcinoma. The porphyrin excretion patterns, in all cases reported, were not consistent with any of the inherited porphyrias, and it is thought that the tumour porphyrin production results from faulty enzyme control.

6. General management is based on the identification and avoidance of all triggering factors (**Fig. 21.10**). Withdrawal from alcohol, prescribed oestrogens, and iron supplements, will, by itself, gradually induce a slow remission, but more active treatment is usually required. Patients should also be advised about sun protection.

    The removal of iron by venesection is, at present, the treatment of choice in PCT: 500 ml of blood is removed, at 2-weekly intervals, until clinical remission or until the haemoglobin falls below 12g/dl. If venesection is contraindicated, low-dose chloroquine is an alternative, and iron-chelating agents such as desferrioxamine can be used for patients on haemodialysis where neither treatment is an option. Beta-carotene has been successfully used to treat patients with the rare erythropoietic porphyria (**Fig. 21.11**).

→ Fig. 21.10
Drugs to be avoided by patients with porphyria.

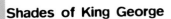

Drugs to be avoided by patients with porphyria	
Sulfonamides	Griseofulvin
Barbiturates	Chloroquine
Glutethimide	Bemigride (only available in USA)
Hydantoins	Oestrogenic substances
Methyldopa (possibly)	Dichloralphenazone

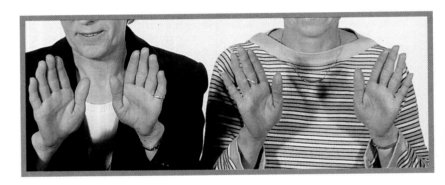

↑ Fig. 21.11
These sisters have the rare erythropoietic porphyria, which remains well controlled on treatment with beta-carotene, hence the orange-coloured palms.

22 | Psoriasis – or not?

Case History

A 74-year-old man had suffered from psoriasis since the age of 20 years. The diagnosis had never been in doubt, and had been confirmed by a dermatologist. The patient's daughter also had psoriasis.

His eruption had varied in severity over the years, but was usually mild and confined to the legs. However, he also had psoriatic arthropathy of the hands, for which he was under the care of a rheumatologist. Radiographs of the hands showed erosive changes in the affected metacarpophalangeal joints (**Fig. 22.1**). Treatment with sulphasalazine had helped this.

Although his rash had become more extensive recently, the patient felt that it was still due to psoriasis, but his rheumatologist disagreed, having detected annular lesions that were thickened and not particularly scaly (**Fig. 22.2**). Skin scrapings were negative for fungi and the patient was referred to the dermatology department for a skin biopsy (**Fig. 22.3**). Later, many of his lesions ulcerated (**Fig. 22.4**).

→ Fig. 22.1
This radiograph shows an asymmetric erosive arthropathy.

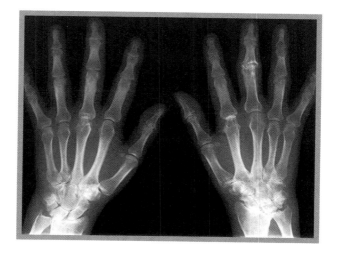

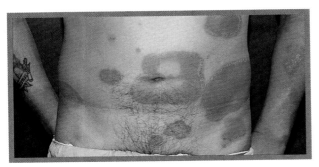

← Fig. 22.2
Annular lesions on the trunk: thickened, barely scaly, and not acceptable as psoriasis.

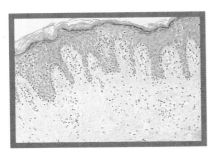

← Fig. 22.3
This condition can produce any pattern of inflammatory skin disease. This biopsy shows lymphocytes peppering the epidermis, where they cause little or no spongiosis. Lymphocytes in the epidermis are larger than those in the dermis (the 'Dolly Parton sign'!).

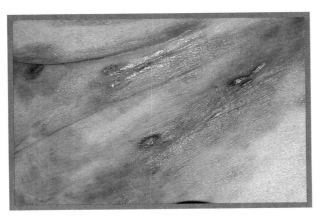

← Fig. 22.4
Multiple ulcers which caused considerable pain.

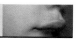

Questions

1. What was the cause of the new skin lesions?
2. What further investigations are needed?
3. How should the condition be treated?

Answers

- The patient now has mycosis fungoides – the most common type of cutaneous T-cell lymphoma. Classically, this passes through three stages, the terminology of which remains difficult. The first (premycotic) stage can look very like psoriasis – hence the term 'parapsoriasis', of which there is a benign type (**Fig. 22.5**) and a premycotic type (**Fig. 22.6**). Poikiloderma (**Fig. 22.7**) – a combination of reticular pigmentation, skin atrophy, and telangiectasia – may also precede mycosis fungoides. Later, lesions pass through the second stage (infiltration) into the third (tumour formation) (**Fig. 22.8**). Progression is usually slow: in one series, the average time from onset to death was 14.5 years.

  In the early, premycotic stage, histology may be nonspecific. Subsequently, a dense infiltrate, composed of atypical, hyperchromatic lymphocytes, with hyperconvoluted nuclei, occupies the papillary dermis. Marker studies show that most of these 'mycosis fungoides cells' belong to the helper subset of lymphocytes and bear the CD4 antigen. They seem to have an affinity for the epidermis (epidermotropism), and some invade it, creating characteristic Pautrier microabscesses (**Fig. 22.9**).

▶ Fig. 22.5
This 'benign' type of parapsoriasis has characteristic yellow–red, finger-like processes that extend round the flanks. It does not turn into mycosis fungoides.

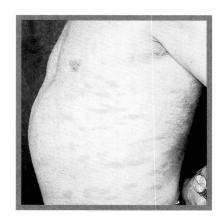

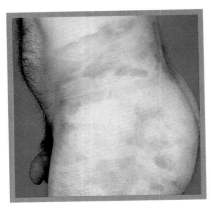

↑ Fig. 22.6
The premycotic type of parapsoriasis can resemble true psoriasis, but some authorities now consider that it is really the patch stage of mycosis fungoides.

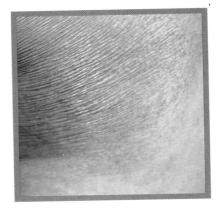

↑ Fig. 22.7
An area of poikiloderma (skin atrophy, telangiectasia, and pigmentation), which may be an expression of mycosis fungoides.

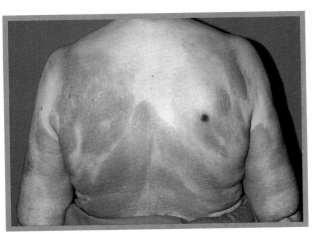

← Fig. 22.8
Large plaques of mycosis fungoides.

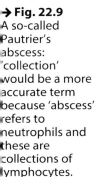

→ Fig. 22.9
A so-called Pautrier's abscess: 'collection' would be a more accurate term because 'abscess' refers to neutrophils and these are collections of lymphocytes.

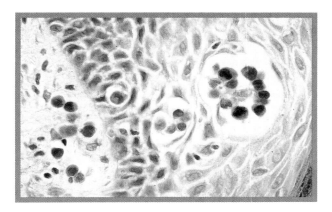

2. In the early stages, when the histology is still not specific, it is particularly important to correlate the clinical with the pathological appearance. Later, immunophenotyping will allow T-cell lymphomas to be differentiated from those involving B cells. Southern blotting can also be used to detect T-cell-receptor gene rearrangements, which in mycosis fungoides reveal a clonal expansion of T cells not seen in normal skin specimens.

The best way of clinically staging mycosis fungoides is still open to debate. However, internal spread, when it occurs, begins with the lymph nodes: any that are palpably enlarged should be biopsied. Other investigations should include a chest X-ray and a full blood count, looking particularly for an overspill of atypical mononuclear cells (Sézary cells) in erythrodermic cases (**Fig. 22.10**).

3. Each patient has to be assessed individually. Highly aggressive treatment may not be appropriate for an elderly patient whose lymphoma is advancing only very slowly.

In the early patch-and-plaque stages of the disease, several treatments can induce useful remissions, although a permanent cure cannot be guaranteed. In one large study, PUVA therapy (**Fig. 22.11**) helped 95% of patients, and cleared 65% completely. Lesions tend to persist in protected sites, such as the flexures. A reasonable alternative is topical nitrogen mustard therapy, although maintenance treatment is needed after clearance has been achieved.

Radiotherapy can be useful in two ways: whole-body electron-beam irradiation is most effective in the absence of thick lesions, as electrons penetrate only to the upper dermis, whereas conventional radiotherapy is of value in dealing with individual tumours. Systemic chemotherapy is usually used in the palliative treatment of advanced disease, and the results may be disappointing.

Extracorporeal photochemophoresis is an interesting new development. Patients are given a psoralen, as in PUVA, and then their white cells are sequestered and passed through a beam of UVA before being reinfused. The results have been most impressive in erythrodermic patients.

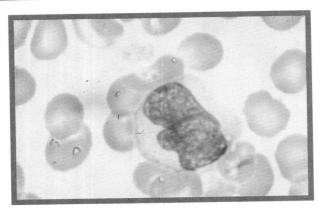

← Fig. 22.10
In erythrodermic mycosis fungoides, atypical mononuclear cells (Sézary cells) may be found in the peripheral blood.

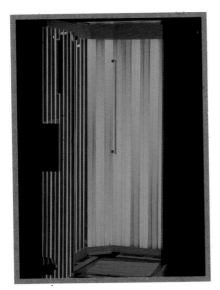

← Fig. 22.11
In PUVA therapy, patients are given oral psoralen and then treated with UVA light in a cabinet like the one shown here.

23 | Feckless and freckled

Case History: Part I

At the age of 12 years, this patient had developed a scaly rash behind one ear (**Fig. 23.1**) and on the nearby scalp (**Fig. 23.2**). His paternal grandfather and his father were thought to have had similar problems. Beta-haemolytic streptococci were isolated on several occasions from splits behind his ears. Soon the rash cropped up also on his feet. Patch testing showed no allergy to his shoes. The correct diagnosis slowly became obvious as the lesions took up a more typical distribution on his elbows and knees (**Fig. 23.3**).

→ Fig. 23.1
The rash below the right ear is still present, 20 years after it first appeared, although the splits within it have become less troublesome.

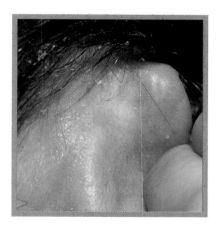

→ Fig. 23.2
Heavy white adherent scaling in the scalp. Note how some scales are stuck to the hairs, lying along their long axes.

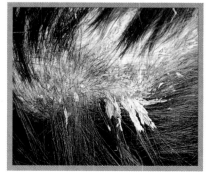

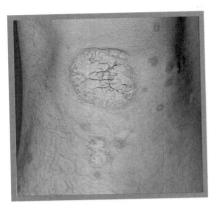

← Fig. 23.3
The eruption in its standard form, on the knee.

Questions

1. What is the correct diagnosis here?
2. Is age at onset important in this condition?
3. Did the streptococcal infection play any part in the worsening of the patient's rash?

Answers

1. This patient has psoriasis. It is not uncommon for psoriasis to start in a child's scalp. Other patterns important in childhood include 'napkin psoriasis' (**Fig. 23.4**), which usually clears quickly but carries a risk of conventional psoriasis developing in later life, and guttate psoriasis (**Fig. 23.5**), a generalised scattering of tiny lesions, sometimes triggered by an acute streptococcal infection.

2. Psoriasis undoubtedly has a strong genetic component, but the different clinical types may represent distinct genetic subpopulations. Evidence for this comes from the differences between psoriasis of early and late onset. Early-onset psoriasis is more strongly associated with human leukocyte antigen (HLA)-CW6 and with a family history of the disease.

3. Streptococcal throat infections are known to trigger guttate psoriasis: in a similar way, recurrent streptococcal infections of a split behind an ear or on the heel (**Fig. 23.6**) may well exacerbate chronic plaque psoriasis. It has also been suggested that having psoriasis confers some selective advantage against streptococcal infections, although the mechanisms involved are still speculative.

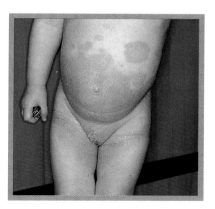

↑ Fig. 23.4.
Napkin psoriasis: a few patches are present outside the napkin area. The condition clears well, but psoriasis may return later in life.

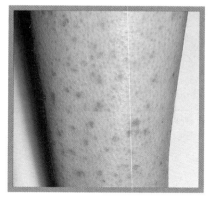

↑ Fig. 23.5
Guttate psoriasis in which the lesions are small but numerous. A common presentation in childhood, and often triggered by streptococcal infections.

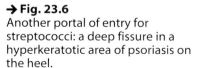

→ Fig. 23.6
Another portal of entry for streptococci: a deep fissure in a hyperkeratotic area of psoriasis on the heel.

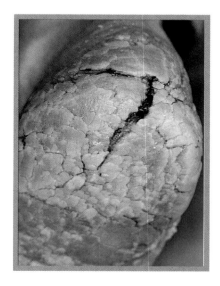

Case History: Part II

The patient's psoriasis remained quiet until he reached the age of 23. By this time, he was smoking 20 cigarettes a day and drinking up to 70 units of alcohol a week. He was not good at treating himself with topical tar or dithranol preparations, although his skin responded well to these on each of several admissions to the dermatology ward. Each admission, however, was followed by a rapid relapse. Consequently, intermittent courses of PUVA therapy were given, and later he received maintenance PUVA therapy. Over the course of the next 7 years, during which he received a total dose of 1450 Joules, his skin developed the changes seen in **Fig. 23.7**.

Questions

1. What are the changes shown in Fig. 23.7?
2. How would you treat this patient now?

Answers

1. These multiple flat, pigmented lesions are PUVA-induced lentigines. They seldom, if ever, transform into malignant melanomas. Indeed, the tumours most commonly induced by prolonged PUVA therapy are Bowen's disease (**Fig. 23.8**) and squamous cell carcinomas, often in those already predisposed to develop them because of earlier exposure to methotrexate, radiotherapy, or excessive sunlight.
2. There are no easy answers here. The patient has shown, on many occasions, that he is unable to use topical treatments successfully. Attendances at a dressings clinic have also been irregular.
    Oral acitretin alone has had little effect, though it did help when given in combination with PUVA. However, we were reluctant to continue with PUVA in view of the already high lifetime cumulative dose.

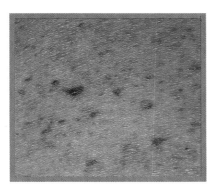

← Fig. 23.7
Irregular dark areas are set against a background of psoriatic erythema.

The next choice might have been methotrexate, but long-term treatment with this carries the risk of cirrhosis of the liver, especially in heavy drinkers. It would have been unsafe to use in this patient as he could not cut down on his alcohol intake.

Instead we used oral cyclosporin therapy, starting at a dose of 3mg/kg/day. The psoriasis cleared well, but relapsed quickly when the treatment was stopped (**Fig. 23.9**), disrupting the patient's life and making him unfit for work. Long-term maintenance therapy is currently keeping the psoriasis under control, but the patient's attendances for tests to monitor renal function are becoming irregular. We no longer measure creatinine clearances routinely in this type of case, but at one stage this patient showed wide fluctuations attributable to the inadequate collection of urine.

Hydroxyurea and azathioprine treatments lie in reserve.

→ Fig. 23.8
An unusually extensive and hyperkeratotic example of Bowen's disease, carrying a high risk of becoming a squamous cell carcinoma.

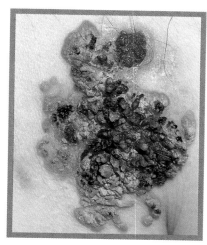

→ Fig. 23.9
Severe relapse after cessation of cyclosporin treatment.

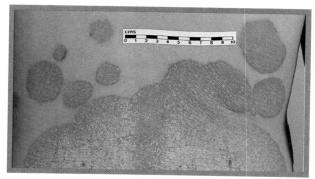

24 | Rings and things

Case History

A 28-year-old woman went on a camping holiday to the Highlands of Scotland in late summer. She was bitten frequently by insects during that week. Four weeks later, a raised red area arose at the site of a presumed bite, and felt like a burn. The redness spread outwards, about 2.5 cm each week, leaving a purplish colour centrally (**Fig. 24.1**). During this time she felt lethargic and vaguely unwell, but had no specific complaints. A number of investigations were performed (**Fig. 24.2**), as well as serological tests, which were negative. Despite these negative tests, she was treated with a specific agent and her rash resolved within 3 weeks.

→ Fig. 24.1
The erythematous ring spread slowly, leaving a purplish discolouration centrally.

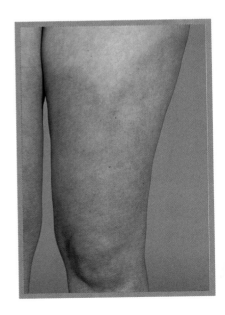

Investigations	
FBC:	Normal
Biochemical screen:	Normal
IgM:	4.3g/l
	(normal=0.4–2.5g/l)
IgG, IgA:	Normal
ANA, complement profile:	Normal

← **Fig. 24.2**
Table of
investigations.

Questions

1. What was the cause of the patient's rash?
2. How would you confirm the diagnosis?
3. What is the differential diagnosis ?
4. How would you treat this condition?

Answers

1.   The rash was due to Lyme disease. This disease was first described in 1977, when a cluster of
children thought to have juvenile rheumatoid arthritis was detected in Lyme, Connecticut.
The rural setting and the identification of erythema chronicum migrans (ECM – **Fig. 24.3**)
as a feature of the illness suggested that it was transmitted by an arthropod. Soon it became
apparent that Lyme disease was a multisystem illness, affecting the skin, nervous system,
heart, and joints. Epidemiological studies of erythema migrans implicated *Ixodes* ticks as the
vector of the disease. In 1982, Burgdorfer isolated a previously unrecognised spirochete (**Fig.
24.4**), now called *Borrelia burgdorferi*, from *I. dammini* ticks (**Fig. 24.5**). Deer (**Fig. 24.6**) are

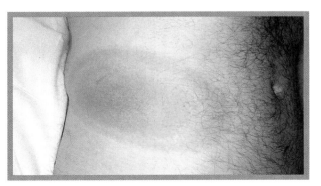

← **Fig. 24.3**
Another example
of erythema
chronicum
migrans due to
Lyme disease.

the preferred host for the adult stage of this tick; however, they have been found on at least 30 types of wild animals and some 50 species of birds. The spirochete was later found in patients with Lyme disease in the United States, and those with erythema migrans or acrodermatitis chronica atrophicans in Europe. This infection resembles syphilis in its multisystem involvement, occurrence in stages, and mimicry of other diseases.

Lyme disease occurs in stages – alone or overlapping.

Stage 1: After injection by the tick, *B. burgdorferi* spreads locally in the skin in 60–80% of patients, and this results in the most distinctive feature of the disease – ECM. The eruption can begin within a few days, or up to 6 weeks later. Erythematous macules or papules appear at the site of the bite, and enlarge: central clearing accompanies peripheral expansion, and the rings commonly reach 15–20 cm in diameter (**Fig. 24.7**). They may be asymptomatic, but are usually associated with a localised burning sensation. Secondary annular lesions are found in some 50% of cases (**Fig. 24.8**). Lymphadenopathy may occur, and excruciating headaches and mild neck stiffness are common, usually lasting only a few hours. The musculoskeletal pain is also transient and typically migratory; debilitating malaise or fatigue may be prominent at this stage. In most patients, these flu-like symptoms subside and the erythema disappears after a few weeks. There may be no symptoms thereafter, or the disease may progress.

A specific IgM response to *B. burgdorferi* occurs within a few weeks, reaching its peak between weeks 3 and 6. This response is frequently associated with polyclonal B-cell activation, elevated total IgM levels, and the presence of cryoprecipitates, circulating immune complexes, and, occasionally, rheumatoid factor, antinuclear antibodies, or anticardiolipin antibodies. All affected tissues are infiltrated with lymphocytes and plentiful plasma cells, and spirochetes show up with silver stains. Mild vasculitis may be seen in several sites, suggesting the presence of immune complexes.

→ Fig. 24.4
Dark field
fluorescence
microscopy
demonstrating
the spirochetes.

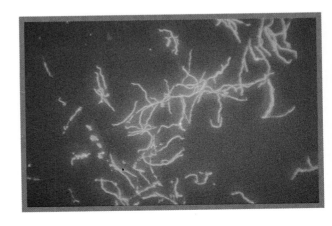

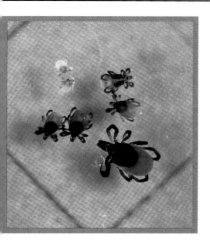

↑ Fig. 24.5
Ixodes ticks in various stages of development.

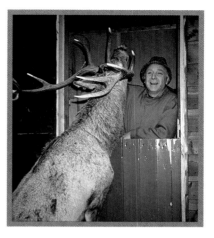

↑ Fig. 24.6
A friendly deer, carrying ticks containing the spirochete of Lyme disease.

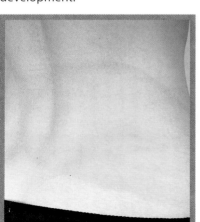

↑ Fig. 24.7
A large and still-expanding area of erythema chronicum migrans.

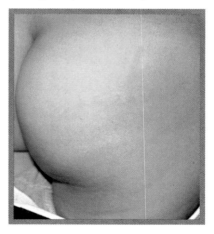

↑ Fig. 24.8
The secondary lesions of erythema chronicum migrans are usually smaller than the primary ones.

Stage 2: *B. burgdorferi* sequesters itself in certain tissues after the original hematogeneous spread; and after weeks or months, as the infection localises, some 20% of patients in the USA develop neurological involvement. Meningitis with a superimposed cranial or peripheral neuropathy is common. The cerebrospinal fluid (CSF) at that stage shows a lymphocytic pleocytosis, often with raised protein but normal glucose levels. In Europe, the first neurological sign is likely to be radicular pain, followed by a pleocytosis in the CSF and lymphocytosis, while meningeal and encephalitic signs are often absent. Stage 2 neurological abnormalities usually last only for a few weeks or months, but may recur or become chronic. Single, red–brown or violaceous nodules and plaques, known as borrelial pseudolymphomas (lymphadenosis benigna cutis), may develop in association with ECM or up to 10 months later.

Several weeks after the onset of the disease, about 5% of patients develop cardiac involvement, which rarely persists for longer than 6 weeks. Fluctuating degrees of atrioventricular heart block are the most common abnormality, and complete heart block, if present, rarely persists for longer than a week. Six months after the onset of the disease, 60% of patients in the USA have begun to have brief attacks of an asymmetric, oligoarticular arthritis, usually of large joints, especially the knee.

Stage 3: Episodes of arthritis become longer during the second and third years of the illness, lasting for months rather than weeks, and chronic arthritis (defined as a year or more of continuous joint inflammation) typically begins in this stage. Joint involvement in European cases is similar, but less frequent. Late neurological sequelae include encephalomyelitis, spastic paraparesis, ataxia, and cranial nerve palsies, but accurate diagnostic tests have yet to be developed.

The best example of prolonged latency in Lyme borreliosis is acrodermatitis chronica atrophicans, a late skin manifestation seen most commonly in European patients. Painless, erythematous, and occasionally infiltrated plaques, appear most commonly on the limbs. The inflammatory phase may persist for several years before leading to skin atrophy.

2. The clinical diagnosis is not difficult if there a history of a tick bite, flu-like illness, and ECM, but few patients recall such a bite and ECM may be absent. Culture and direct visualisation of the *B. burgdorferi* is difficult and takes time. However, the polymerase chain reaction can be used to amplify DNA fragments and produce a rapid diagnosis. The diagnosis may also be based on the presence of IgM or Ig G antibodies to *B. burgdorferi*, using immunofluorescence or enzyme-linked immunosorbent assay (ELISA). With ELISA, cross-reaction may occur with other borrelial infections, and occasionally with connective tissue disease and treponemal infections. ELISA is the most commonly used test, but positive reactions are low in stage 1 disease (about 25%). Antibody responses may be minimised by early antibiotic therapy, although progressive disease may still occur. When the result is still in doubt, immunoblotting can be used to increase sensitivity, but not necessarily specificity, of the test. Still greater sensitivity can be achieved with a two-step ELISA test.

3. The wide range of possible presentations makes the recognition of Lyme disease difficult. The condition is probably now overdiagnosed as a result of media attention. Late neurological complications remain the greatest diagnostic problem. More common is the patient with vague symptoms, such as headache, musculoskeletal pain, and fatigue, which can be confused with fibromyalgia and chronic fatigue syndrome.

The differential diagnosis of ECM includes erythema annulare centrifugum, in which scaling forms on the trailing edge of the expanding annular erythema (**Fig. 24.9**). This feature helps to distinguish it from dermatophyte infections, in which scale forms at the leading edge. Granuloma annulare should be considered, but has a papular margin, progresses very slowly, and is often violaceous (**Fig. 24.10**). The annular lesions of mycosis fungoides are more infiltrated and psoriasis-like.

4. It is still debated whether patients bitten by ticks in areas endemic for Lyme disease should be treated if clinical signs of infection are absent. However, the treatment of early disease (stage 1) prevents the progression of symptoms and stops the *Borrelia* organisms reaching sanctuary sites. Commonly used antibiotics include penicillin V, amoxycillin, doxycycline, tetracycline, minocycline, and azithromycin, for 5–12 days. A few patients will progress to stage 2 disease whatever the treatment. Patients with stage 2 and 3 disease require prolonged oral or intravenous antibiotics, or both. Many trials confirm that the third-generation cephalosporins are superior to penicillin for carditis, arthritis, acrodermatitis chronica atrophicans (ACA), and neurological disease.

▶ Fig. 24.9
In erythema annulare centrifugum, scaling is found on the trailing edge of the ring.

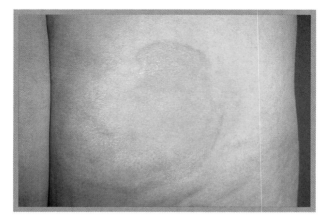

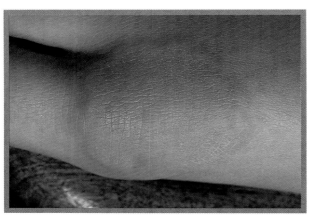

← **Fig. 24.10**
The rings of granuloma annulare have a papular margin and expand slowly.

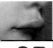

25 | Dangerous swellings

Case History

A woman aged 40 years, had a 15-year history of intermittent swellings, which had appeared with increasing frequency on her feet, hands, and genital area. The most recent episode had affected her face (**Fig. 25.1**) and throat, and had followed a visit to the dentist. No other triggering factors had been identified.

Each episode of swelling had lasted about 48 hours (**Fig. 25.2a–c**), and had not been accompanied by itching or any eruption elsewhere. No obstruction to breathing had ever occurred, even when her face had been swollen.

Her attacks were occasionally associated with abdominal colic, but this feature was more marked in a younger sister, who suffered regularly from unexplained abdominal pains and who had even been admitted to hospital on three occasions with suspected appendicitis. Some of her sister's episodes of abdominal pain had been accompanied by swellings on the limbs.

Neither sibling was convinced that antihistamines or systemic corticosteroids, oral or intravenous, had been of any help.

▶ Fig. 25.1
An example of gross swelling of the upper lip.

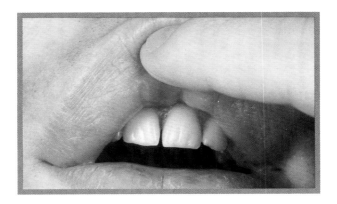

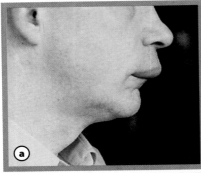

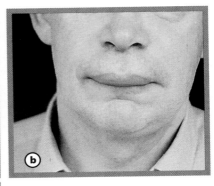

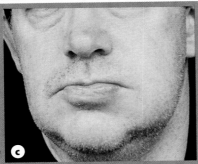

← ↑**Fig. 25.2**
Another patient with the same
condition whose appearance
changed dramatically according to
whether the upper (**a** and **b**) or
lower (**c**) lip was affected.

Questions

1. What is the most likely diagnosis here?
2. How should this patient and her sister be investigated?
3. What risks does the condition carry?
4. How should it be treated?

Answers

1. This patient has the rare hereditary form of angioedema. Unlike the far commoner condition
    of nonfamilial angioedema, the familial type is not associated with itchy urticarial lesions
    elsewhere (**Fig. 25.3**). Inheritance is as an autosomal dominant trait. Remember that other
    conditions such as contact eczema (**Fig. 25.4**) and even dermatomyositis (**Fig. 25.5**) can cause
    swollen eyelids. Swollen lips, also, can have other causes (**Fig. 25.6**). Always ask about possible
    drug causes (**Fig. 25.7**), particularly salicylates (aspirin) and other mast-cell histamine releasers
    such as codeine phosphate .

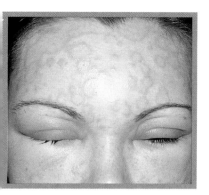

↑ Fig. 25.3
Gross swelling of the eyelids: the presence of itchy urticarial wheals elsewhere on the face makes it unlikely that this is the familial type of angioedema.

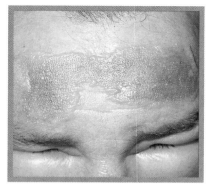

↑ Fig. 25.4
Allergic contact dermatitis: this reaction to an antiseptic applied to the forehead is accompanied by a massive swelling of the lids of both eyes.

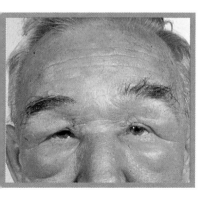

↑ Fig. 25.5
In dermatomyositis, the periorbital oedema may be mistaken for angioedema.

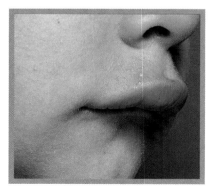

↑ Fig. 25.6
Granulomatous cheilitis: permanent swelling of the lips may be a feature of Crohn's disease. Rarely it is due to an allergy to a constituent of toothpaste.

2. There are two types of hereditary angioedema (HAE), which are clinically indistinguishable. Both are based on abnormalities in the gene coding for C_1 esterase inhibitor, lying on chromosome 11q. The C_1 esterase inhibitor is a glycoprotein with a molecular weight of 105 kDa. When attached to activated C_1 esterase, it blocks complement activation.

In HAE type I, which accounts for about 85% of patients, abnormally low levels of the inhibitor are found: in the rarer HAE type II, levels of the inhibitor, as measured immunologically, seem normal or even high, but the inhibitor fails to function normally.

The laboratory diagnosis of HAE is based on immunochemical assays of the C_1 esterase inhibitor and C_4 levels. If both are decreased (as in this patient and her sister – **Fig. 25.8**), the HAE is of type I. If the C_1 esterase inhibitor level is normal, but the C_4 level is low, type II is likely, and a functional analysis should be performed.

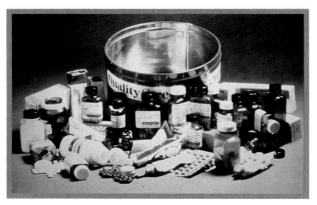

← Fig. 25.7
One patient's cache of drugs, not including the aspirin found in her handbag.

Investigations			
Test	Patient	Sister	Normal range
C_1 inhibitor activity	14%	17%	75–125% HNP
C_4	<0.10g/l	0.09g/l	0.12–0.30g/l

↑ Fig. 25.8
Table of tests.

3. HAE is rare but important – up to 35% of untreated sufferers die from laryngeal obstruction. This is an emergency, and epinephrine is of less value than in the nonhereditary type (**Fig. 25.9**). A patent airway has to be established as quickly as possible. Thereafter, the most important emergency treatment of respiratory obstruction is with C1 inhibitor – either in the form of a concentrate, if available, or freshly reconstituted, freeze-dried whole plasma. Attacks of angioedema often seem to be triggered by trauma, notably by dental extractions and surgery: C1 inhibitor concentrate can also be used prophylactically before such procedures are undertaken. Finally, acute episodes can be helped by esterase inhibitors, such as trasylol and ε-amino capnoic acid.

Patients should always carry a card stating the diagnosis and outlining possible emergency treaments. Other complications include abdominal crises (with severe abdominal pain and watery diarrhoea).

4. The management of acute episodes is outlined in the answer to Question 3. It is worth mentioning that systemic antihistamines and corticosteroids are usually of little value.

Possible long-term treatments include danazol, a weak androgen that increases the synthesis of the C1 inhibitor, but it may have androgenic side effects in women. The use of tranexamic acid can also be considered.

➜ Fig. 25.9
The needle of this minijet syringe, which contains epiniphrine, will even pierce eans. Patients usually use an out-of-date syringe and practice on an orange first.

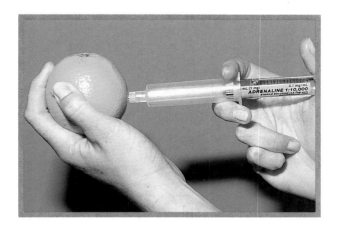

INDEX

Numbers are page numbers.

A

acetretin, 89, 142
  adverse effects, 90
acne, 37
acrodermatitis chronica atrophicans, 146, 148
acrodermatitis enteropathica, 18
actinic reticuloid *see* chronic actinic dermatitis
acute febrile neutrophilic dermatosis *see*
          Sweet's syndrome
acyclovir, 60
adenocarcinoma, metatastic, 18
Addison's disease, 71, 72
adipocyte necrosis, 9
AIDS, 73
  Kaposi's sarcoma associated, 117
  prognosis, 125
  syphilis associated, 121–2
  treatment, 125
aldolase, 4
alendronate, 60
allergic contact dermatitis, 153
ε-amino caproic acid, 155
amoxycillin, 149
Amsler chart, 29, 30
angiocentric immunoproliferative lymphoma
          (AIL), 95
angular stomatitis, 136
antibiotics, 60, 95, 149
anticardiolipin antibody, 29
antihistamines, 41
antimalarials, 29
antineutrophil cytoplasmic antibody (ANCA), 17, 93
  classic (c-ANCA), 17
  Goodpasture type (IgM-ANCA), 17
  Henoch–Schönlein type (IgA-ANCA), 17
  perinuclear (p-ANCA), 17
  Sweet's syndrome, 17
antiphospholipid syndrome, 29
α1-antitrypsin, 11
antituberculosis drugs, 84
aphthous ulcers, 18
Aspergillus fumigatus, 11
aspirin, 17
autoimmune polyendocrinopathy–candidiasis–
          ectodermal–dysplasia (candidiasis
          endocrinopathy syndrome), 74
azathioprine, 52, 60, 143
azelaic acid, 22

B

bacillary angiomatosis (BA), 121
barbiturates, 48, 132
Bartonella henselae, 121
basal cell carcinoma (BCC), 93, 94

Behçet's syndrome, 18
benzodiazepines, 96
beta-carotene, 131
Borrelia burgdorferei, 145–6, 148
Bowen's disease, 142, 143

C

C1 inhibitor, 155
calcinosis, 5
cancer, temporal relationship to dermatomyositis, 6
Candida albicans, 73
candidiasis endocrinopathy syndrome (auto
          immune polyendocrinopathy–candidiasis
          dysplasia), 74
capillaritis, 35
captopril, 48
carbamazepine, 95-6
catheters, 64-5
cephalosporins, 149
chemotherapy, 118
chloroquine, 131, 132
chlorpromazine, 107
chronic active dermatitis (actinic reticuloid), 97–103
  clinical features, 99
  investigations, 98, 102
  treatment, 103
chronic active hepatitis, 41
chronic fatigue syndrome, 149
chronic mucocutaneous candidiasis, 69–74
  angular stomatitis, 69
  Candida albicans infection, 73
  candidal pseudohyphae/spores, 73
  diagnosis, 73
  mouth scrapings, 73
  nail lesions, 70–1, 74
  tongue lesion, 69, 70
  treatment, 74
chrysanthemum allergy, 97, 102
clindamycin, 22
clonidine, 48
confetti-like hypopigmentation, 22
connective tissue disease, panniculitis associated, 11
contact urticaria, 67
corticosteroids, 17, 41, 42
creatine phosphokinase (CPK), 4
Crohn's disease, 18
  granulomatous cheilitis, 153
  pyoderma gangrenosum, 114
  Sweet's syndrome associated, 17, 18
cryoglobulinemia, 27
cryptococcosis, 124
Cryptococcus neoformans, 124
cutis marmorata, 27
cyclophosphamide, 42, 60
cyclosporin, 60, 115, 143

D

Danazol, 155
dapsone, 115
Darier's disease, 85–90
  acantholytic keratinocytes, 88
  clinical features, 87
  complications, 89
    cutaneous, 89
    neuropsychiatric, 89
    salivary gland swelling, 89
  differential diagnosis 87
  dyskeratotic cells, 88
  histological features, 87
  inheritance, 87
  lithium effect, 90
  papules, 85, 86, 87
    warty, 88
  photosensitivity, 99
  round bodies (corps ronds), 89
  treatment, 89–90
  yellowish scaling of scalp/forehead, 86
delusional parasitosis, 78
  treatment, 79
dermatitis herpetiformis, 106
dermatomyositis (DM), 1–6, 153
  age groups, 6
  autoantibodies, 5
  calcinosis, 5
  carcinoma associated, 5, 6
  cardiac involvement, 5
  esophageal dysmotility, 5
  Gottron's papules, 2, 3
  investigations, 3, 4–5
    creatine phosphokinase (CP), 4
    electromyography, 4
    magnetic resonance imaging, 4
    muscle biopsy, 4
    skin biopsy, 5
  lung disease, 5
  malignancy associated, 5
  muscles affected, 5
  vasculitis, 5
desferrioxamine, 131
diabetes mellitus, 11, 107, 129
  steroid-induced, 60
diarrhoea, traveller with, 13–18
digitate dermatosis see parapsoriasis
digoxin, 60
dimethyl sulfoxide, 64
diphenylhydantoin, 53
discoid eczema, 27
DM see dermatomyositis
Dolly Parton sign, 134
doxycycline, 121, 149
drug eruptions, 18
dusky erythema, 1–2

E

eczema, discoid, 27
electromyography, 4
EM see erythema multiforme
emollients, 41
enzyme-linked immunosorbent assay (ELISA), 148
eosinophilic folliculitis, 124
epidermolysis bullosa acquisita, 18
Epidermophyton floccosum, 122
epidermotropism, 135
erythema annulare centrifugum, 149
erythema chronicum migrans, 146, 147
erythema induratum (nodular vasculitis), 10
erythema multiforme (EM), 17, 49–54, 119
  clinical features, 51–2
  complications, 54
    death from, 54
  drug associated, 53
  haemorrhagic crusting, 50
  herpes (HSV) associated, 52, 54
    keatinocyte nuclear changes, 54
  investigations, 49, 51
  management, 52
  mycoplasma associated, 53
  major, 54
  precipitating factors, 52–3
  skin biopsy, 54
  treatment, 52, 54
erythema nodosum, 9, 10, 11, 18
erythrodermic mycosis fungoides, 138
erythromycin, 121
espundia (South American leishmaniasis), 95
esterase inhibitors, 155
ethambutol, 84
etretinate, 89
European Standard Battery of Contact Allergens, 67, 68
extracorporeal photochemophoresis, 137
eyelid swelling, 1

F

fibromyalgia, 149
fifth cranial nerve's spinal tract, 96
fixed drug eruption, 64, 65
fluconazole, 122
fluoxetine, 60
Foscavir (foscarnet sodium), 120
freeze-dried whole plasma, 155
frusemide, 99

G

giant cells, 53
gingivitis, 18
glomerulonephritis, mesangioproliferative, 34
Gottron's papules, 2, 3
graft-versus-host disease, 39

granuloma, 81–4
  biopsy, 83
  chest radiograph, 81
  clinical features, 82–3
  differential diagnosis, 83
  lynphohistiocytic infiltrate, 81
  midline, 95
  sarcoid, 83
granuloma annulare, 11, 12, 150
granulomatous cheilitis, 153
grey face, man with, 19–23
griseofulvin, 42, 101, 132
'grog blossom', 21
gumma, 93

H

HAE *see* hereditary angioedema
Hailey–Hailey disease, 87
hairy leukoplakia, 73
HCV *see* hepatitis C virus
heliotrope plants, 3
haemopoietic malignancies, 112
Henoch–Schönlein purpura (HSP), 36
hepatitis, chronic active, 41
hepatitis C virus (HCV), 41
  skin diseases associated, 41
hepatocellular carcinoma, 131
hereditary angioedema (HAE), 151–5
  acute episodes, 155
  investigations, 154
  management, 155
  types, 154
herpes labialis, 49
herpes simplex, 99, 119–20
histidyl tRNA synthetase antibody, 5
HIV infection, 47, 73, 119–22
Hodgkin's disease, 107
human leukocyte antigen (HLA)-CW6, 140
human herpesvirus-8, 118
hydantoins, 132
hydrochlorothiazide, 100
hydroquinone, 22
hydroxychloroquine, 29
hydroxyurea, 143
hypersensitivity, 67
  delayed, 67, 68
  immediate, 67
hypoglycemia, oral, 74

I

IgA, 36
IgG, 36
  autoantibodies, 58–9
IgM, 36
immunoglobulin infusion, 60
immunofluorescence, 148

immunoreactants, 114
indomethacin, 17
infarction, CT brain scan, 26
inositol, 90
interferon, 118
interleukin-2, 118
interstitial fibrosis, 5
isoniazid, 84
itching *see* pruritus
itraconazole, 74, 124

K

Kaposi's sarcoma (KS), 116–25
  African, 117
  AIDS associated, 117
  classic, 117
  clinical features, 117–18
  HIV infection, 118–21
  post-renal transplantation, 117
keloid, 82
ketoconazole, 122
ketotifen, 48
Klebsiella rhinoscleromatis, 95
Köebner phenomenon, 37, 39

L

latex, soft rubber, 64
Leishmania, 83
leishmaniasis, South American (espundia), 95
leprosy, 83
leukemia, 18
  Sweet's syndrome associated, 18
leukocytoclastic (allergic, necrotizing) vasculitis, 31–6
  immune-complex-mediated, 36
  investigations, 32
    renal, 33, 34
  prognosis, 36
  purpura, 31, 32
  treatment, 36
lichenoid eruption, drug caused, 41
lichen planus (LP), 37–42
  aetiology, 39
  bullous, 39, 40
  clinical features, 39–40
  differential diagnosis, 41
  histology, 41
  hypergranulosis, 42
  hypertrophic, 39
  Köebner phenomenon, 37, 39
  liver disease associated, 41
  nail changes, 38, 40–1
  treatment, 41–2
  Wickham's striae, 39
lithium, 90
livedo reticularis, 25, 27
LP *see* lichen planus

lupus erythematosus (LE), 3, 11, 27
  acute cutaneous, 3
  discoid, 27
lupus pernio, 95
lupus profundus, 11
lupus vulgaris, 83–4
  antituberculosis regimen, 84
  squamous carcinoma development, 83
  untreated, 83
Lyme disease, 144–50
  complications, 148
  deer, 146, 147
  treatment, 149
lymphoma, 18, 59
  cutaneous, 112

M

malignancy, association with age, 6
melasma, 22, 23
methotrexate, 143
mthyldopa 132
methylprednisolone, 60
metronidazole, 21–2, 48, 124
minocycline, 21, 115, 149
monocycline-induced hyperpigmentation, 20–1
monoclonal gammopathy, 115
molluscum contagiosum, 120–1
morphea, 11
mucocutaneous candidiasis, 122
'muddy skin' syndrome, 20, 21
muscle calcinosis, 5
Mycobacterium avium intracellulare (MAI), 122
myelodysplasia, 18
Mycoplasma pneumoniae, 53
mycosis fungoides 133–8
  annular lesions, 134
  clinical features, 135–7
  Dolly Parton sign, 134
  erosive arthropathy, 133
  inflammatory skin disease, 134
  patch stage, 136
  Pautrier microabscesses, 135, 137
  plaques, 136
  treatment, 137, 138
  ulcers, 134
myeloma, 18
myeloproliferative disorders, 18

N

nevus of Ota, 21
nails
  'half and half', 104
  longitudinal brown lines, 71
  notched, 85–90
  striped, 69–74
  thumb nail dystrophy, 70

nasal ulceration, 91–6
necrobiosis lipoidica diabeticorum, 11
necrotizing fasciitis, 113
necrotizing vasculitis, 18
neuroleptics, 79
neutrophilic dermatoses of myeloproliferative
    diseases, 114
Nikolsky sign, 57
nitrogen mustard, 137
nodular vasculitis (erythema induratum), 10

O

ochronosis, 22
oestrogenic substances, 132
ovarian carcinoma, 18

P

palmar erythema, 105
pancreatitis, chronic, 7
panniculitis, 7–11
  connective tissue disease associated, 11
  histopathology, 9–10
  infections, 11
  investigations, 8
  lobular, 9
  metabolic, 11
  pancreatic, 7–11
  physical 11
  septal, 9
  thrombophlebitis associated, 11
paraproteinemias, 121
parapsoriasis (digitate dermatosis), 47
  benign, 135
  premycotic type, 136
patch test, 102
PCT *see* porphyria cutanea tarda,
pellagra, 18
pemphigoid, 57 58, 59
pemphigus, 87
  erythematosus, 57, 58
  foliaceus, 57
pemphigus vulgaris, 55–61
  acantholytic cells, 58
  clinical features, 57
  death from, 60, 61
  histology, 58
  IgG autoantibodies, 58
  immunofluorescence of biopsy specimen, 58, 59
  mouth ulcers, 55
  neck erosions, 56
  Nikolsky sign, 57
  polymorphic skin lesions, 59
  skin biopsy, 56
  stomatitis, 59
  treatment, 60
    side effects, 60

penicillin derivatives, 53
penicillin V, 149
penile lesions, 63–7
  fixed drug eruptions, 64
  fungal, 64
  oedema, 67
  psoriasis, 64, 65
  seborrheic dermatitis, 64
percutaneous transhepatic cholangiogram, 108
periorbital oedema, 1, 3
periungual erythema, 1
posterythema revealed telangiectasis (PERT), 22
petechiae, 35
PG *see* pyoderma gangrenosum
phenylbutazone, 53
phenytoin, 74
pigmented purpuric dermatosis, 35
pimozide, 79
pityriasisform reactions, drug-induced, 48
pityriasis rosea, 43–8, 119
  biopsy, 47
  clinical features, 45
  differential diagnosis, 47–8
  herald patch, 45
  histology, 47
  investigations, 44
  meaning of 'pityriasis', 45
  prodromal symptoms, 45
  rash, 43
    oval lesions, 46
    scaly collarettes, 46
    T-shirt distribution, 44, 45
  scaling rim, 43
  treatment, 47
photochemotherapy (PUVA), 42
photosensitivity, 99–103
  causes, 99
  drug-induced, 99–101
phototoxic reaction, 101
phytophotodermatitis, 99
pityrosporum folliculitis, 122
pityrosporum yeasts, 123
plakoglobin, 58
plasmapheresis, 60
pneumonia, aspiration, 5
polyarteritis nodosa, 27
  HIV infection associated, 4
polycythemia, 106
polycythemia rubra vera, 113
polymorphic light eruption, 27, 99, 100
polymyositis, 5
porphyria, 128
  action spectrum, 130
  drugs to be avoided, 132
porphyria cutanea tarda (PCT), 126–32
  alcohol associated, 128
  clinical features, 129

factors, 128
familial, 129
hepatocellular carcinoma associated, 131
hepatitis C (HCV) markers, 131
infection associated, 41
management, 131
skin biopsy, 131
posterythema revealed telangiectasia (PERT), 22
posterior inferior cerebellar artery syndrome, 96
postherpetic neuralgia, 120
potassium hydroxide, 64
potassium iodide, 10, 17
prednisolone, 60, 113, 115
prostatic carcinoma, 18
proteinuria, pain and, 31–6
prurigo, HIV infection associated, 41
prurigo nodularis, 75–9
  treatment, 79
pruritus (itching), 104–9
  conditions causing, 107
  investigation, 106, 108–9
    percutaneous transhepatic cholangiography, 109
  treatment, 103
pseudoporphyria, 131
psoriasis, 83, 133, 139–43
  adherent scalp scaling, 139
  guttate 48, 141
  napkin, 141
  penile, 64, 65
  PUVA-induced lentigines, 142
  streptococcal throat infection triggered, 140,141
  treatment, 90
purpura, 18, 32
  painful, 31
  solar, 35
PUVA (photochemotherapy), 42
pyoderma gangrenosum (PG), 110–15
  associated diseases, 112
  atypical 18, 114
  bullous, 115
  clinical features, 112–13
  histology, 114
  investigation, 111
  monoclonal gammopathy associated, 115
  pathogenesis, 114
  treatment, 115
pyrazinamide, 84

R
radiotherapy, 118, 137
ranitidine, 60
rash stroke, 24–9
RAST test, 67
rectal mucosa, granulomatous infiltration, 15
Reiter's syndrome, 125
retinoids, 89, 90
rheumatoid arthritis, 18, 110, 112

rheumatoid-like arthritis, 112
rhinophyma, 23
rhinoscleroma, 95, 96
rifampicin, 84
rosacea, 21–2, 27
  rhinophyma associated, 23
  treatment, 21–2
rubber
  chemical allergens, 68
  contact allergy, 64, 66–7

S

sarcoidosis, 11, 83
scabies, 106
scurvy, 18
seborrheic dermatitis, 122, 123
  penile lesion, 64
severe combined deficiency disease, 73
Sjögren's syndrome, 18
skin calcinosis, 5
skin patch testing, 67
skin 'splinters', 75–9
SLE *see* systemic lupus erythematosus
squamous cell carcinoma, 83, 93
Staphylococcus aureus, 89, 121
steroids,
  fluorinated, 21
  intralesional, 115
  panniculitis due to, 11
  systemic, 10, 11
  topical 17, 41, 42, 52
Stevens–Johnson syndrome, 52
stomatitis, 18
streaky rash, 1–6
subacute cutaneous lupus erythematosus, (SCLE) 27
sulfonamides, 53, 132
sunscreens, 102
  tinted, 103
suppurative folliculitis, 114
Sweet's syndrome (acute febrile neutrophilic
        dermatosis), 13–16
  annular erythematous plaques, 16
  arcuate lesion, 16
  associated conditions, 17–18
    secondary to treatment, 18
  atypical, 18, 114
  clinical features, 16–17
  diarrhoea, 13–16
  endothelial cells, 15
  granulomatous inflammation of rectal mucosa, 15
  histology, 17
  investigations, 14
  neurophil infiltration in papillary dermis, 15, 16
  oedematous plaques, 13
  pathogenesis, 114
  pseudovesicular papules, 16
  skin biopsy, 15

subepidermal vesiculation, 15
  treatment, 17
  tumid plaque, 14
  yersinia infection, 17
syphilis, 121–2, 119
  congenital, 93, 94
  gumma, 93
  secondary, 47
  shin pain, 47
syringomyelia, 96
systemic lupus erythematosus (SLE), 27–9
  anticardiolipin antibody, 29
  butterfly rash, 28
  chronic mucocutaneous candidiasis associated, 73
  discoid, 27, 28
    IgG deposition at dermoepidermal junction, 28
    treatment, 29
  erythematous polycyclic lesion, 30
  prognosis, 27
  treatment, 29
systemic sclerosis, 3

T

telangiectasia, 1, 3, 22
tendon calcinosis, 5
terbinafine, 122
terfenadine, 74
testicular carcinoma, 18
testosterone, 107
tetracycline, 149
thrombocytopenia, 27
thrombophlebitis, 11
thymoma, 59, 73
tinea corporis, 48
tinea pedis, 122
tinea versicolor, 122
tranexamic acid, 155
transient acantholytic dermatosis, 87
Treponema pallidum, 121
triamcinolone, 42
Trichophyton rubrum, 122
trigeminal nucleus, conditions affecting, 96
trigeminal trophic syndrome, 91–6
  clinical features, 92
  differential diagnosis, 93–5
  management, 95–6
  skin biopsy, 91
tuberculosis, 83–4
  chest radiography, 81
  nodular vasculitis associated, 10
Tzanck smear, 53, 119

U

ulcerative colitis, 18
ulcers, 55–61
urticaria, 17, 155

contact, 67
HIV infection associated 41
uvethon-Y screens, 103

V
varicella-zoster virus (VZV), 120
vasculitis, 24
  HIV infection associated, 41
  leukocytoclastic *see* leukocytoclastic (allergic,
    necrotizing) vasculitis,
  livedo, 34
  septic, 34
vitamin A deficiency, 89
vulvovaginitis, chronic, 73

W
warfarin, 74
Wegener's granulamotosis (WG), 93, 94
Wickham's striae, 39
winter-itch, 106

X
xeroderma pigmentosum, 99

Z
zidovudine, 118, 119